Gerald Pichler
Franz Fazekas

Apallic syndrome

Gerald Pichler
Franz Fazekas

Apallic syndrome

Frequency and care provision in Austria

ScienciaScripts

Imprint
Any brand names and product names mentioned in this book are subject to trademark, brand or patent protection and are trademarks or registered trademarks of their respective holders. The use of brand names, product names, common names, trade names, product descriptions etc. even without a particular marking in this work is in no way to be construed to mean that such names may be regarded as unrestricted in respect of trademark and brand protection legislation and could thus be used by anyone.

Cover image: www.ingimage.com

This book is a translation from the original published under ISBN 978-3-639-88744-0.

Publisher:
Sciencia Scripts
is a trademark of
Dodo Books Indian Ocean Ltd. and OmniScriptum S.R.L publishing group

120 High Road, East Finchley, London, N2 9ED, United Kingdom
Str. Armeneasca 28/1, office 1, Chisinau MD-2012, Republic of Moldova, Europe
Managing Directors: Ieva Konstantinova, Victoria Ursu
info@omniscriptum.com

Printed at: see last page
ISBN: 978-620-9-79370-7

TABLE OF CONTENTS

CHAPTER 1

Introduction

'Apallic syndrome' (persistent vegetative state) is one of the most severe neurological conditions. The primary feature is the absence of conscious awareness of one's own person and the environment. Furthermore, those affected suffer from pronounced motor and sensory deficits, are unable to communicate and are incontinent. The patients' inability to express their needs, as well as frequent bronchopulmonary and urogenital infections and autonomic dysfunction, demand a high degree of professionalism and flexibility from carers.

In most cases, it is acute cardiopulmonary or acute primary cerebral events, such as haemorrhages or trauma, that tear those affected and their relatives away from their normal lives. Those affected can no longer look after their own affairs and are now completely dependent on outside help.

The question of how to optimise further care for these patients, as well as the issue of withholding treatment and euthanasia—which has already been discussed on numerous occasions in other countries due to specific circumstances—will certainly pose a major challenge for our society in the future. Patients in a minimally conscious state (MCS) and patients with locked-in syndrome (LIS) are similarly severely affected individuals. However, recognising a minimally conscious state is not always straightforward in practice.

Accurate epidemiological data form the basis for any considerations and planning aimed at optimising patient care. Of particular importance here are the number of new cases (incidence) as well as the total number of people affected (prevalence). The latter depends on the incidence and the chronicity (survival duration).

The first part of this book outlines the general fundamentals. These include the clinical description of the disease course (remission phases), pathophysiology, diagnosis, differential diagnosis and the prognosis of this condition. It then presents the incidence data for apallic syndrome in the province of Styria and discusses these findings in the context of the current literature. At the end of the book, the care structure in Austria is examined and the model of optimised care in the province of Styria is described as a representative example.

CHAPTER 2

History and Definition

Historically, it is worth noting that the first patient with apallic syndrome was presumably described as early as the late 19th century by Rosenblath (1899) as *a 'remarkable case of concussion'*. The patient was a 16-year-old tightrope walker who had fallen from a height of several metres and survived for eight months in a *"strange state of consciousness"*. This persistent disturbance of consciousness is likely to have corresponded to apallic syndrome. Since then, this clinical picture has entered the literature under various synonyms (Table 1).

Table 1

Synonyms for apallic syndrome

Rosenblath	Remarkable case of concussion	1899
Kretschmer	Apallic syndrome	1940
French	Prolonged unconsciousness	1952
Fischgold	Post-comatose hypertonic stupor	1959
Sutter	Post-traumatic catatonia	1959
Jellinger	Protracted form of post-traumatic encephalopathy	1963
Barley blight	Traumatic apallic syndrome	1967
Jennet, Plum	Vegetative state	1972

The term **'apallic syndrome'** (AS) was first introduced into the literature by Kretschmer (1940). The term is derived from the Latin 'a pallium' (i.e. absence of the mantle or cerebral cortex) and refers to the loss of function of the cerebral cortex. Kretschmer had already pointed out that, despite its severe neurological symptoms, apallic syndrome is a functional disorder of the cerebral cortex that can resolve. He described the clinical symptoms, their pathophysiological aetiology and the course of remission in a 30-year-old female patient who had suffered from panencephalitis. She exhibited primitive motor patterns, mass movements ( ), signs of extrapyramidal motor damage, autonomic disturbances, and a lack of responsiveness despite her eyes opening intermittently. As the syndrome resolved, emotional reactions first emerged and primitive motor function began to diminish. Following increasing engagement with the environment, the final presentation consisted of spastic tetraparesis with cerebellar symptoms, affective incontinence, and signs of a psychotic syndrome. The patient ultimately died shortly after discharge, reportedly as a result of an epileptic seizure. A second patient following a brain injury was consulted solely to confirm the clinical symptoms. Investigations such as computed tomography (CT) and magnetic resonance imaging (MRI), which would have allowed visualisation of the accompanying morphological changes, were not available at the time of the initial description.

The first detailed description of apallic syndrome was published by Gerstenbrand (1967) in the form of a monograph. In this work, which provided a detailed account of 74 patients with apallic syndrome of traumatic aetiology, he was able to distinguish between an *initial stage*, a *transitional stage* leading to apallic syndrome, the *full-blown form of apallic syndrome*, and eight *stages of remission*. The clinical symptoms he described, their progression, the pathophysiology, and also the therapeutic approaches are still regarded worldwide today as the basis for the diagnosis and treatment of this severe neurological condition. According to current knowledge, the use of the term 'apallic syndrome' is problematic because this condition does not involve a complete separation of the cortex from the brainstem (a-pallium), and the term therefore corresponds neither functionally nor anatomically.

In the English-speaking world, the clinical picture only found its way into the literature at a later date. Jennett and Plum (1972) proposed the term **'persistent vegetative state'** (PVS), which, despite its vague usage and negative connotations ('vegetating'; 'vegetative' = plant-like), has become widely established in the international literature. In accordance with a recommendation by the Multi-Society Task Force on PVS (1994) of the , this term applies once the condition has persisted for a period of one month. If the clinical picture persists unchanged thereafter, the use of the term **"permanent vegetative state"** was recommended for patients following non-traumatic brain injury for a period exceeding 3 months, or following traumatic brain injury for a period exceeding 12 months. The term "vegetable", derived in some cases abusively from "vegetative", and the aspect of permanence conveyed by the addition of "permanent" led to calls, both in public debate and in religious circles, for the introduction of a less discriminatory term. Jennet et al. (1997) addressed this by proposing that the terms "persistent" and "permanent" be avoided so as not to unnecessarily imply the aspect of "permanence".

In German-speaking countries, the term **'Wachkoma'** is frequently used instead of 'apallic syndrome'. This is derived from the French term "coma vigile" and very effectively describes the discrepancy—clearly recognisable even to laypeople—between "being awake" (eyes open) and the lack of responsiveness (coma) of the affected person. Although this term is not a medical one, it is, for the reasons mentioned, well established in both public and political discourse in German-speaking countries.

Due to the problems outlined regarding the naming of this severe cerebral dysfunction, a *"European Working Group"* proposed the term

'unresponsive wakefulness syndrome' (UWS) (Laureys et al. 2010). The authors justify this by stating that the term is very neutral and accurately describes the key clinical signs, such as the lack of responsiveness and the presence of wakefulness.

Finally, it is worth mentioning a term that has become established in the literature to describe people with minimal conscious activity. The *"Aspen Neurobehavioural Conference Workgroup"* defined this condition as the **"minimally conscious state"** (Giacino et al. 2002). This largely corresponds to the clinical picture of the "early remission phases" described by Gerstenbrand.A precise differentiation regarding the level of consciousness therefore seems very important, as in numerous countries and various other cultural contexts, the duration of therapy and the treatment resources made available depend significantly on this differentiation.

CHAPTER 3

Clinical description

3.1 Initial stage and transitional stage to apallic syndrome

The initial stage following severe acute brain injury usually progresses in clearly distinguishable phases and is temporally associated with the loss of cerebral function. A decisive factor here is the intracranial volume increase that almost always occurs in severe acute brain injury, leading on the one hand to the displacement of brain structures and on the other to increased pressure. This increase in volume is often caused by cerebral oedema or an extra- or intracerebral haematoma. In severe cases, this initially leads to herniation at the falx cerebri and later to clinically significant tentorial uncal herniation or, in the worst-case scenario, to foraminous herniation, i.e. entrapment in the foramen magnum. The more or less rapid collapse of the cerebral regulatory systems and their control over the brainstem centres governing motor and autonomic functions, as well as the failure of the afferent systems and the ascending reticular formation, trigger a gradual loss of consciousness accompanied by disinhibition of the brainstem-controlled anti-gravity motor functions as well as the autonomic regulatory centres of the brainstem. There is an increasing extension posture of the extremities with extension synergies, as well as disturbances in respiratory and circulatory function. Clinically, the symptoms of acute midbrain syndrome are now evident. This may occur secondarily as a result of tentorial herniation, presenting with a medial course (central herniation) or a lateral course (uncal herniation). In central herniation, the medial temporal lobe, pressed into the tentorium, exerts bilateral pressure on the midbrain. In uncal herniation, unilateral pressure is exerted by the protruding medial temporal lobe on the brainstem, pressing it against the sharp contralateral edge of the tentorium. Following acute primary damage to the midbrain, the initial stage progresses rapidly through phases of varying distinctness ( ) and is almost always followed by an apallic syndrome. If the supratentorial or infratentorial volume increase persists and foraminous herniation occurs, an acute bulbar brain syndrome may develop, which very often proves fatal.

It should be noted that, whilst the phases of acute midbrain syndrome and acute bulbar brain syndrome are in principle clinically well-defined, analgosedation is mandatory in the current intensive care management of these patients. As a result of the additional 'central depression' caused by this, the functions of the brainstem regulatory centres are also reduced. The patients are placed on mechanical ventilation and require circulatory monitoring. Consequently, the fluid transitions between these stages can no longer be precisely distinguished clinically.

It is assumed that the transition to the full-blown apallic syndrome takes between 14 and 21 days (Gerstenbrand, 1967). This assumption is also consistent with the guidelines of the Royal College of Physicians (Bates, 2005), according to which the diagnosis of a 'vegetative state' should be made no earlier than 4 weeks after the acute event.

3.2 Symptoms of the full-blown apallic syndrome

Historically, Kretschmer described apallic syndrome in 1940 (pp. 577–578) as follows: *'The patients lie there with their eyes open... Despite being awake, the patients are unable to speak, recognise things or perform meaningful, learned actions. In contrast, certain basic vegetative functions, such as swallowing, are preserved. Furthermore, known early deep reflexes, such as the sucking reflex or the grasping reflex, become prominent."*

The symptoms of apallic syndrome following acute severe brain damage, but also in the terminal stage of a progressive cerebral disease, ultimately correspond to the complete failure of all cerebral functions, with a decline in the level of central nervous system function to the meso-diencephalic level (Gerstenbrand, 1967). The functional cause is therefore the impairment of all tract systems connecting the midbrain with the thalamus and the cerebral cortex or the brainstem. The main symptom is wakefulness (open eyes) with a preserved fatigue-dependent sleep-wake rhythm and the inability to recognise the environment and make contact with it. All cerebral functions of voluntary motor control, as well as all sensory feedback systems, are impaired. There is a lack of appropriate responses to external stimuli. Autonomic reactions occur in response to external or internal pain stimuli. Brainstem functions may be largely preserved or even enhanced. As a possible increase in visceral functions, tachycardia, hypertension, hyperthermia, increased excretion and heightened sebum, sweat and saliva production may occur. There is also complete faecal and urinary incontinence. Patients are usually in a flexed-extended posture of the limbs and body. Primitive motor reflexes and frontal movement patterns, such as the grasping reflex, sucking reflex and smacking, as well as postural and positioning reflexes, are also frequently present (Aichner et al. 1982). These manifestations may also be misinterpreted as a response or an attempt to make contact. Finally, severe dysphagia should be mentioned, which is why the insertion of a PEG tube and often also a tracheostomy tube is necessary. At this point, it is important to highlight the need to distinguish apallic syndrome from classic locked-in syndrome (LIS). In LIS, the patient is completely paralysed, with the exception of vertical eye movements and eyelid movements, and is thus 'trapped' within their own body whilst remaining conscious. The symptoms of the full clinical picture of apallic syndrome are summarised in Table 2.

Table 2

Apallic syndrome in its full-blown form – clinical symptoms

- No conscious awareness of oneself or the environment
- Sleep-wake cycle controlled by fatigue
- No gaze fixation, no eye-tracking movements
- No adequate response to external stimuli (e.g. visual, auditory, tactile)
- Autonomic reactions and undirected, uncoordinated movements in response to pain
- Absence of voluntary motor function, flexion-extension posture of the limbs
- Increased muscle tone
- Primitive motor patterns (e.g. oral reflexes, grasping reflex)
- Absence of verbal utterances, lack of language comprehension
- Autonomic dysregulation

Secondary and tertiary complications such as contractures, ossifications, polyneuropathies, pressure ulcers of the skin or even vertebro-spinal changes frequently develop over time.

3.3 Remission phases of apallic syndrome

Many patients do not remain in the full-blown stage of apallic syndrome but show improvement in their clinical condition. Gerstenbrand (1967) identifies eight phases (remission phases) that flow seamlessly into one another within the context of this potential improvement (see Table 3).

Table 3

Remission phases according to Gerstenbrand

Phase 1	Phase of primitive psychomotor function
Phase 2	Reaching phase
Phase 3	Pre-Klüver-Bucy syndrome
Stage 4	Klüver-Bucy syndrome
Phase 5	Post-Klüver-Bucy syndrome
Phase 6	Korsakoff's syndrome
Phase 7	Wernicke's syndrome
Phase 8	Amnestic syndrome

In the first two phases, there is a shift from a sleep-wake state determined by fatigue to a sleep-wake rhythm dependent on the time of day. Following the onset of visual fixation, visual tracking of objects within the visual field becomes the most important clinical sign from phase 2 onwards.

In phases 3–5, specific symptoms of Klüver–Bucy syndrome come to the fore (Gerstenbrand et al. 1983). These involve grasping objects and a subsequent tendency to put them in the mouth, chew them and swallow them, without, however, recognising the object. A further symptom of Klüver-Bucy syndrome is an increasing interest in the genitals, which is acted upon without any sense of shame. The disinhibition of the limbic system explains not only these sexual behavioural abnormalities but also an increasing emotional disinhibition. In phase 5, purposeful movements can be performed to some extent in response to prompts. Focal neurological deficits are now becoming increasingly apparent. Primitive vocalisations give way to the first attempts at speech, and oral feeding can usually be initiated. Korsakoff's syndrome is the primary feature of the 6th remission phase. Emotions and feelings become increasingly attuned to the specific situational context. Global attention is increasingly followed by a differentiated recognition of people and objects. Purposeful voluntary movements, whether spontaneous or in response to verbal prompts, occur more frequently. Following phase 7, which is characterised by amnestic disorders, the 8th remission phase presents symptoms of a diffuse organic psychosyndrome. In principle, a significant recovery of health is possible from every phase; however, most of these patients only reach what is known as an 'early remission stage' (phases 1–3). This condition is equivalent to the Anglo-American 'minimally conscious state' (see 2.2.5). In any case, a rapid diagnosis, intensive neurological rehabilitation and follow-up treatment in a suitably specialised neurological care unit for patients in a persistent vegetative state appear to be key elements for an optimal recovery. Over the last two decades, it has increasingly been pointed out that the diagnosis of 'full-blown apallic syndrome' is often not correctly made. Diagnostic errors can result from limited experience in assessing this relatively rare clinical picture and from the varied and sometimes confusing terminology (Monti et al. 2010). Often, it is the onset of gaze fixation or eye-tracking movements in those affected that are not recognised, or only recognised at a later stage (Schnakers et al. 2009). Both the observations of the care team and feedback from relatives are important in this regard. All authors recommend the use of a validated assessment scale in addition to the clinical examination.

3.4 Deficit stage of apallic syndrome

The clinical symptoms of apallic syndrome depend on the location and intensity of the primary lesion (traumatic, hypoxic, encephalitic, vascular) as well as on irreversible secondary damage and complications (Gerstenbrand, 1967; von Wild et al. 2007). These complications include, for example, polyneuropathy, myelopathy, hydrocephalus, malnutrition, avitaminosis, periarticular ossifications, joint contractures (Zhuber et al. 1977), pressure points on peripheral nerves (Mamoli et al. 1977), as well as pressure ulcers and recurrent bronchopulmonary and urogenital infections.

If there is no remission of the full-blown apallic syndrome, the term 'permanent' is used in the English-language literature to describe this stage of the condition. There are varying timeframes regarding when a "persistent vegetative state" should be classified as a "permanent vegetative state". The Multi-Society Task Force on PVS (1994) defined this time limit as 1 year for patients with a traumatic aetiology and 3 months for those with a non-traumatic cause. The Royal College of Physicians (Bates, 2005) recommends a time limit of at least 6 months for the latter group. Finally, the development of the so-called "bed rest syndrome" should be mentioned. This can develop as a result of patients remaining in a horizontal position for too long. A lack of stimulation in the vestibular system and in the area of gravity receptors—the most important stimulatory factor—leads to functional disorders of the proprioceptive system. Pathophysiologically, this 'bed rest syndrome' is comparable to 'astronaut syndrome' (Artner et al. 1993). The symptoms consist of primary muscle atrophy, polyneuropathy, disorders of the posterior column systems (pseudotabes), as well as thalamic disorders and a reduction in the activation of the 'ascending reticular activating system', which is also important for attention.

3.5 Minimally conscious state

The term "minimally conscious state" (MCS) was introduced into the literature by Giacino et al. (2002) and refers to patients with clearly perceptible behaviour suggesting conscious awareness of both themselves and their environment . Clinically, as already mentioned, this corresponds to the early remission phases following Gerstenbrand's disease. Further improvement in the state of consciousness of this patient group is possible and also more likely than in individuals with the full-blown apallic syndrome. However, it is also possible for patients to remain in the MCS state permanently, although there is currently no consensus on the definition of a permanent MCS. The diagnostic criteria for MCS, translated into German and made available to the collaborating partners in this study, are listed in the appendix.

CHAPTER 4

Pathophysiology

Kretschmer (1940) had already emphasised the loss of all cerebral functions in the first description of apallic symptoms. The functional level of the human brain is reduced to the mesodiencephalic level (Gerstenbrand, 1967; von Wild et al. 2007). With the loss of the cerebral cortex's control systems, the autonomic regulatory centres of the brainstem take over. Patients presenting with the full picture of apallic syndrome are unable to process stimuli from the environment; all capacity for memory retention has been lost. Furthermore, all voluntary motor control functions and sensory perception are completely lost. However, perception of external and internal stimuli does occur at the brainstem level. Historically, there have been very different explanatory approaches to the functional pathophysiology of consciousness (Latin: conscientia; 'awareness or conscience'). According to a current definition, consciousness is the awareness of the self and its environment and describes the degree to which an organism perceives stimuli and is awake (Jellinger, 2009).

According to Butler et al. (2005), consciousness encompasses areas of attention, internal sensation, sensory perception, planning, motor function, volition, language and self-awareness, and is regarded as a necessary prerequisite for complex cognition. A concept for the functional-anatomical substrate of consciousness was outlined by Dehaene et al. (2006). According to this, there is a functional hierarchy comprising three functional circuits that interact dynamically. The first level is a subcortical network that controls arousal and wakefulness. It comprises the mesencephalic reticular formation and its projections to the thalamus. The second level comprises a mixed cortical-subcortical network with diffuse projections via the thalamus, the hypothalamus and the brainstem. As the final level, the authors identified a predominantly cortical network between association areas in the posterior parietal and dorsolateral frontal cortex, the prefrontal cortex ( ) and the primary sensory cortex.

The complete failure of cerebral function with apallic symptoms can be explained by the various neuropathological changes and their differing lesion patterns. A primary lesion in the midbrain or brainstem region can also trigger a functional failure of the cerebrum (Gerstenbrand, 1967). Similarly, a functional breakdown of the cerebral cortex can be triggered by diffuse or multi-focal cortical lesions and by pronounced damage to the white matter. Lesions in the relay centres of the thalamus and the basal ganglia are further potential causes of apallic syndrome. This was unfortunately demonstrated following initial unsuccessful stereotactic surgeries for the treatment of extrapyramidal disorders.

In addition to the primary mechanisms already described, secondary mechanisms of damage must also be mentioned. In this context, the concept of the penumbra and the periepicentre is of crucial importance. With rapid and appropriate treatment, it is possible to restore brain tissue in the penumbra that is initially only partially damaged, whereas in the umbra, the epicentre, no restoration is possible due to the primary destruction of the brain tissue. All measures of acute treatment are therefore aimed at minimising irreversible permanent damage to the penumbra tissue as much as possible. It is therefore understandable that patients with traumatic brain injury may suffer additional hypoxic deficits when intracranial pressure rises, or that it is these secondary hypoxic defects that lead to the development of apallic syndrome in the first place.

In traumatic apallic syndrome, the primary damage to brain tissue caused at the moment of the traumatic impact – due to its location, direction and intensity (open or closed head injury) – has a decisive influence on the resulting structural damage and thus on the subsequent course of the condition. In addition, reference should also be made here once again to the potentially irreversible secondary damage in the penumbra, as well as to secondary damage in the form of diffuse and regional lesions, which may be triggered in part by accompanying cerebral oedema. In traumatic apallic syndrome, highly diverse lesion patterns are observed (Gerstenbrand, 1967; Jellinger, 1968 & 1977; Jellinger et al. 1963). In most cases, there is marked damage in the bilateral medullary layers of the cerebral hemispheres. Furthermore, anatomical and functional disruptions of the tract systems may occur as a result of 'diffuse axonal injury' (Adams et al. 1982). These are caused by acceleration and deceleration forces, as well as rotational forces. Areas with varying tissue density (e.g. the transition from the cortex to the white matter) and other brain regions that are particularly vulnerable to the forces acting upon them (e.g. the corpus callosum and brainstem) are considered sites of predilection. Ultimately, however, it is usually not the primary mechanical damage to the axons that is responsible for the functional deficits, but rather a biochemical cascade that sets in after hours or days. This leads to calcium influx into the cell and ultimately to the activation of phospholipases and proteolytic enzymes, which eventually results in separation from the axon and cell death.

In apallic syndrome, secondary damage is also caused as a consequence of tentorial herniation. This is due to mass shifts resulting from cerebral oedema, subdural or epidural haemorrhages. Accompanying hypoxic damage may also lead to additional changes in the diencephalon.

In cases of hypoxic causes of apallic syndrome (cardiac arrest, near-drowning, strangulation, etc.), extensive laminar necrosis of the cerebral cortex may occur in a diffuse, regional or extensive multifocal form. Other areas particularly predisposed to hypoxia include the hippocampus, the brainstem and the subcortical nuclei, with the thalamus and striatum being primarily affected (Jellinger, 1994; Kinney & Samuels, 1994). In hypoxia-induced apallic syndrome, lesions are also frequently found in the arterial border zones of the parasagittal parieto-occipital cortex, in the basal ganglia ( ) and in areas that exhibit particular vulnerability in relation to the vascular supply. Overall, the hypoxic-ischaemic lesion pattern primarily affects the thalamus, with the territory supplied by the thalamo-perforate artery and the thalamo-geniculate artery being particularly at risk due to compression of the posterior cerebral artery as a result of tentorial herniation. Finally, a third hypoxic-ischaemic lesion pattern consists of diffuse damage to the medullary layers and hypoxic leukoencephalopathy with bilateral demyelination lesions or necrosis (Kinney & Samuels, 1994).

Similar changes are observed in apallic patients following carbon monoxide or nitrogen oxide poisoning, or following exogenous intoxication. Here too, there is diffuse damage to the medulla or changes in the form of hypoxic leukoencephalopathy with extensive demyelination lesions or necrosis. According to Jellinger (1994), the histological features of brain tissue lesions include the loss of neurons, synapses and glial cells, as well as signs of damage or shear injuries to axons. Substantive damage arises from hypoxia or anoxia, from intoxication, but also from secondary inflammatory and immune processes.

In apallic syndrome, focal and diffuse structural damage mainly affects the cerebral cortex and the medulla. Focal lesions often also affect the diencephalon and the upper brainstem. The Klüver-Bucy syndrome is primarily caused by damage to the limbic system, which may also serve as a partial explanation for the symptoms of the Korsakoff phase.

CHAPTER 5

Diagnosis

The diagnosis of apallic syndrome is based primarily on clinical examination. In addition to the clinical neurological examination, scales should also be used. In specialised research centres, attempts are also made to obtain evidence of conscious activity in patients using functional magnetic resonance imaging (fMRI), electroencephalography or event-related potentials, which is of enormous importance, particularly in the differential diagnosis of the 'minimally conscious state'. However, these additional investigations often have limitations in terms of their routine applicability, which is why they are usually only used for research purposes.

The main clinical neurological criteria are the lack of conscious perception of the environment and of one's own person, the absence of adequate and reproducible responses to visual, auditory, olfactory and tactile stimuli, as well as the lack of language comprehension and the inability to express oneself. For further details on clinical symptoms, please refer to Chapter 2.2 (Clinical Description). Of particular importance in this context is the fact that any behaviours exhibited by patients that suggest conscious awareness are often not observable throughout the entire course of the day, but only intermittently. It is particularly difficult to differentiate between emerging voluntary motor function and reflex-induced movement patterns and primitive motor reflexes. It must also be borne in mind that patients in a minimally conscious state usually have only very limited ability to indicate this.

The timing of diagnosis is not uniformly specified in the literature. The data are particularly inconsistent regarding the transition from a persistent vegetative state to a permanent vegetative state. However, there is agreement that the diagnosis of 'apallic syndrome' (vegetative state) should not be made until at least four weeks have elapsed following the acute event. A further prerequisite is that extreme care must be taken to ensure that patients are not sedated at the time of examination, are free of fever, and that metabolic imbalances have been largely corrected. In addition to all these points, the examiner's experience is of great importance.

There are currently a number of validated scales that can be used for the diagnosis and differential diagnosis of apallic syndrome. The paper by Seel et al. (2010) provides a good overview of these. The rationale for selecting the 'Coma Recovery Scale revised' (CRS-R) for this study is set out in Chapter 3.5.2. An extract from the manual, translated into German, is included in the Appendix.

CHAPTER 6

Differential diagnoses

In each patient, there is a different type of damage to the areas and pathways in the brain responsible for consciousness, or a central nervous system suppression of the associated functions of varying duration and severity caused by intensive care medications. Consequently, particularly in the acute phase, it is not always easy to distinguish apallic syndrome from other serious brain dysfunctions or from a prolonged coma. Added to this are possible psychiatric conditions that may mimic severe cerebral dysfunction or that may co-exist with central nervous system disorders in affected individuals. Clinical presentations such as akinetic mutism, dissociative stupor or catatonic stupor may lead to such differential diagnostic considerations.

Misdiagnoses of patients in a minimally conscious state are very common. This is demonstrated by retrospective clinical studies (Andrews et al. 1996; Childs et al. 1993; Gill-Thwaites & Munday, 2004) as well as study results in which well-validated scales were additionally used (Gill-Thwaites, 1997; Schnakers et al. 2009). The reported incidence of misdiagnosis in these studies ranges from 18% to 43%. The authors cite a lack of experience in dealing with this relatively rare patient group, inconsistent terminology, and varying points of diagnosis as key factors contributing to misdiagnosis. In a retrospective study, Andrews et al. (1996) found that many misdiagnosed patients with minimal consciousness were unable to respond to external stimuli as expected due to their severe physical impairment. Sensory impairments, and in particular visual impairments, are also frequently the cause of incorrect diagnoses (Childs et al. 1993). Electrophysiological investigations are increasingly enabling these hidden aspects of consciousness in MCS patients to be better recorded. In future, these capabilities could also be utilised to establish communication via brain-computer interfaces (BCI) . Initial promising results, using auditory event-related potentials (p300), were reported by the research group at Graz University of Technology in collaboration with the Albert Schweitzer Clinic in Graz (Müller-Putz et al. 2012).

Functional magnetic resonance imaging (fMRI) and electroencephalography may also become increasingly important for the differential diagnosis between full-blown apallic syndrome and the early stages of remission (minimally conscious state). For example, Schabus et al. (2011) investigated whether there were differences in brainwave recordings between patients with apallic syndrome and those in a minimally conscious state regarding the processing of spoken semantic word pairs and antonyms. The results showed that this was possible in patients in a minimally conscious state, but not in patients clinically classified as apallic. The same research group also found that, unlike patients with full-blown apallic syndrome, MCS patients were able to process a visually presented grasping movement of the hand at the sensory and premotor levels (Lechinger et al. 2013). The study by Monti et al. (2010) attracted considerable attention. The researchers reported evidence that some patients classified as being in a 'vegetative state' were able to consciously imagine playing tennis and walking through their house. This conclusion was drawn from activation patterns in fMRI, which, although attenuated in patients in the 'vegetative state', were similar to those observed in healthy subjects. One patient, who had also been classified as being in a 'vegetative state' during preliminary examinations, subsequently answered 5 out of 6 questions about his personal life correctly using the power of thought. This study impressively demonstrated how difficult it is in individual cases to detect covert behaviour solely through clinical assessment.

In this context, it is also noted that secondary, treatable complications, such as hydrocephalus, can lead to a regression in disease remission. If these conditions are not detected early and treated, they could also unnecessarily influence the diagnosis of the condition and lead to a diagnosis of full-blown apallic syndrome in an MCS patient (Monti et al. 2009).

Finally, the important differential diagnosis of 'locked-in syndrome' is described. Locked-in syndrome is a clinical picture of similar severity to apallic syndrome, but which, in its classic course (Bauer et al. 1979; Bauer et al. 1983; Plum & Posner, 1972), differs fundamentally in that the patient retains consciousness. Consequently, an accurate diagnosis and differentiation between these two clinical presentations is of particular importance. The patient with classic locked-in syndrome is completely paralysed, apart from the ability to open their eyes and make vertical eye movements; however, the sensory systems remain intact. Hearing and vision are preserved, as are the sensation of pain and the perception of the surroundings. The term was introduced into the literature by Plum and Posner (1972). However, locked-in syndrome was first described more than 100 years earlier by Alexandre Dumas in the novel 'The Count of Monte Cristo'. The character described there, the father of one of Edmond Dantès's enemies, is said to have 'his soul imprisoned within his own body'. He is described as completely powerless, yet with 'living eyes'. Sight and hearing were the two sensory functions that maintained contact with the outside world. The sufferer could also communicate with those around him by blinking. This description is particularly remarkable, as Alexandre Dumas was a writer and not a doctor. In isolated cases, 'apparent death' can presumably also be cited as a historical medical model of locked-in syndrome in its acute form.

This is the condition of the human fate feared for centuries: being buried alive, although there may be other causes for this besides locked-in syndrome. The most prominent victim is considered to be the Russian writer Nikolai Vasilyevich Gogol, whose skeleton was found in a completely contorted position during exhumation after five years. It was assumed that this resulted from his desperate attempt to free himself from the grave. The symptoms of classic locked-in syndrome are summarised in Table 4.

Table 4

Symptoms of locked-in syndrome

- Loss of all voluntary motor function
- Vertical eye movements and opening of the eyes possible
- Swallowing difficulties
- Spontaneous breathing maintained
- Consciousness undisturbed; able to perceive what is happening in the surroundings
- No verbal communication, but ability to understand speech

Pathophysiologically, locked-in syndrome involves bilateral damage to the ventral pons, with disruption of the corticospinal and corticobulbar tracts. The somatosensory and ascending reticular systems remain functional. Furthermore, the tectum of the brainstem is not affected, which is why vertical eye movements are possible. The causes of locked-in syndrome include ischaemic strokes, haemorrhages, injuries and inflammatory conditions.

In the acute stage, locked-in syndrome may occur in combination with acute midbrain syndrome, and later also with apallic syndrome. This combination is referred to as 'locked-in plus'. In a relatively high percentage of cases, locked-in syndrome shows remission, which can sometimes lead to a high degree of independence for patients, but usually still presents with severe deficits.

CHAPTER 7

Prognosis

Predicting the likelihood of acute brain damage progressing to apallic syndrome, and forecasting the temporal course of this clinical picture, remains difficult despite all the additional investigations currently available in the acute phase. Partial remission is, in principle, possible in all patients following severe acute brain damage and acute intoxication. However, a very large number die within the first few years following the acute event. In a follow-up study, Higashi et al. (1981) demonstrated that within the first 5 years following the acute event, 73% of all patients with apallic syndrome had died, whilst only approximately 10% achieved partial remission of the full clinical picture. Of the total of 110 patients in this study, communication was established with 3 patients, and 2 individuals achieved independence in their daily activities by the 5-year follow-up.

The most comprehensive prognostic data were published by the 'Multi-Society Task Force on PVS' (1994). Of the total of 754 documented patients, 43% showed signs of consciousness after one year, 34% died and only 23% remained in a state of apallic syndrome with the full clinical picture. The longer the condition persisted, the less likely remission was (after 6 months, only 13%). Patients with a traumatic aetiology improved more frequently, and children showed marginally better outcomes than adults.

Overall, three factors appear to be of particular importance for the prognosis of apallic syndrome (Monti et al. 2010). One factor is the duration of the apallic syndrome, with remission becoming increasingly unlikely as the duration of the condition increases. Furthermore, the age of the patient plays an important role, as the capacity for neuroplasticity decreases with increasing age. In addition, older patients increasingly have co-morbidities , which in turn may limit the likelihood of remission. The cause of the disease was confirmed in this study as a third important prognostic factor. It should be noted here that patients with a traumatic cause generally have a better chance of recovery. In summary, the probability of remission is lowest in older patients following hypoxic brain damage that occurred a long time ago.

In traumatic apallic syndrome, severe structural damage—which can be diagnosed using magnetic resonance imaging—carries a poor prognosis. In particular, damage to the corpus callosum and the dorsolateral brainstem indicates a poor prognosis (Kampfl et al. 1998). Particularly in cases of hypoxic aetiology, a prognosis regarding survival and, above all, the quality of survival can usually be established after a few weeks to months through a thorough clinical examination, regular follow-up checks and additional diagnostic tests. These additional investigations include magnetic resonance imaging (MRI), electroencephalography (EEG), somatosensory evoked potentials (SSEPs) and laboratory parameters (e.g. neuron-specific enolase).

Passing through the early remission phases and entering the Klüver-Bucy phase is a favourable prognostic sign for further regression of apallic syndrome (Formisano et al. 1995). It should be particularly emphasised that significant clinical improvements are still possible even years later (Andrews, 1993).

If the underlying cause of apallic syndrome is a progressive neurodegenerative disease or a chronic metabolic disorder (e.g. hepatic encephalopathy due to liver cirrhosis), the possibility of remission does not, in principle, exist.

CHAPTER 8

Incidence Survey Methodology

8.1 Study objective

Due to the increasing ability in recent years to visualise covert behaviour using technical investigative methods (e.g. fMRI), both public and scientific interest in the topic of 'apallic syndrome' has grown. This has led to increasing pressure on political decision-makers, who bear primary responsibility for planning care for these patients. A well-structured care system allows, on the one hand, the patients' rehabilitation potential to be utilised to the full and, on the other hand, provides the best possible relief for the family environment. As the clinical picture of apallic syndrome represents an 'ethical grey area', the continuous accumulation of scientifically sound knowledge is of particular importance. The basis for optimising the care structure is accurate data on the prevalence of the condition and an inventory of current care options in Styria. The aim of this study is therefore to determine the incidence of apallic syndrome in Styria and to identify which facilities patients were admitted to and for how long they remained in inpatient care at those facilities. These data can be incorporated into future planning within Styria's 'Regional Health Structure Plan' (RSG). It is reasonable to assume that, given the similar conditions within the healthcare system, these data can be extrapolated to the whole of Austria and will also provide valuable insights beyond national borders.

8.2 Study type

The present study is a prospective cohort study.

In this case, it is an incidence study, i.e. a population-based study of a cohort without a control group. This study design is used to provide information on the distribution and frequency of occurrence of health-related characteristics or diseases. The advantage of prospective studies compared to retrospective studies is that the type, scope and quality of the data to be collected are considered in advance, can be ideally adapted to the precisely defined objectives, and can be continuously reviewed and monitored during the study.

Cohort studies are a type of observational study. This means that researchers observe events from a passive position without intervening in the process itself. These studies are therefore also well-suited to tracking the progression of diseases.

Advantages of cohort studies:

The cohort study examines the population of interest directly, and the group is not selected beforehand, or only to a limited extent, by inclusion and exclusion criteria, and is thus researched in a 'real-life situation'. The advantage of this 'real-life' research is the associated high external validity. Due to the usually large number of study participants, these studies are well suited to identifying even rare diseases. Cohort studies whose participants represent an entire population can be used to collect epidemiological data, such as incidence rates.

Disadvantages of cohort studies:

One disadvantage of this type of study is that they often take a very long time. This becomes problematic if environmental conditions change during a long observation period (e.g. new diagnostic criteria or a change in collaborating partners). Consequently, in cohort studies it is important to ensure reliable participation through careful management and monitoring of the study. This type of study is particularly labour-intensive and expensive, especially with large study populations.

In cohort studies involving the formation of comparison groups, it must be assumed that systematic differences exist within the comparison groups. These systematic errors are referred to as selection bias. This can lead to factors – which are not actually the subject of the investigation but are nevertheless associated with the outcome – obscuring the relationships under investigation. These factors are called confounders. As no comparison groups were formed in the present study, the factors described (selection bias and confounders) are mitigated. Nevertheless, particular attention was paid to these potentially interfering factors during the planning and definition of the inclusion and exclusion criteria.

8.3 Study population and duration

As the primary objective was to determine the incidence of apallic syndrome in the adult population, the study population was defined as all persons aged 18 and over registered as having their main residence in Styria. According to current data from 'Statistik Austria', this represented a population of 1,010,164 people during the study period (2012).

A detailed breakdown by age group, excluding those under 18 years of age, was also taken from the Statistik Austria database and is presented in Table 5.

Table 5

Study population and age groups

Age	Number
18 years	14,147
19 years	14,944
20–24 years	78,223
25–29 years	78,891
30–44 years	252,757
45–59 years	272,272
60–74 years	190,763
75 years and over	108,167
	1,010,164 total

Internet source: http://statcube.at

A period of one year was chosen for the study. It was anticipated that, over such a period, participation from all centres would be sufficiently high and that a sufficient number of patients would be registered at to provide valid data for the main question of the study. The study ran from 1 December 2011 to 30 November 2012.

8.4 Study centres

Given the expected low incidence of apallic syndrome in absolute terms, the utmost importance was attached to the need for the most comprehensive possible recording of all new cases with their main residence in Styria. To this end, cooperation was sought with all institutions that might care for patients in both the acute and post-acute phases of apallic syndrome. These include all neurological departments, all acute care hospitals with intensive care or monitoring wards, and all Styrian neurorehabilitation clinics (Table 11). The majority of these institutions are managed by KAGES (Styrian Hospitals Association). The Medical Directorate of KAGES kindly agreed to support the study. This greatly facilitated the recruitment and coordination of the study centres.

In the border regions of Styria, where the geographical accessibility of acute care hospitals would have made it conceivable to admit affected patients to a neighbouring federal state, all relevant district branches of the Red Cross were contacted by telephone. These were the district branches in Tamsweg, Güssing and Wolfsberg. Based on the feedback received from these district offices, the likelihood of such seriously ill patients being admitted to a neighbouring federal state appeared remote. Consequently, the additional participation of hospitals in neighbouring federal states was deemed unnecessary. Although eligible study patients are not treated in rehabilitation clinics during the acute phase of the illness, all Styrian rehabilitation facilities were also invited to participate in the study. The reasoning behind this was, on the one hand, to provide a double safeguard for data collection, and on the other hand, to account for the possibility that a patient with their main residence in the Styrian Health Authority ( ) might have suffered the acute event in another federal state or even abroad. As these patients may be transferred back to their home federal state, at least for neurorehabilitation, cooperation with the rehabilitation clinics in the study increased the likelihood of registering these patients as well.

The selection of study centres to be recruited for the study was primarily based on the Hospital Compass (www.spitalskompass.at) and the Rehabilitation Compass (www.rehakompass.at) of the ÖBIG (Austrian Federal Institute for Health). Further additional information was obtained through collaboration with KAGES and following direct contact with the respective institutions.

Initially, all directors or medical directors of the selected study centres were contacted. For KAGES hospitals, the initial contact and invitation to participate in the study were made via the KAGES Executive Board, and for the University Hospital of Graz via the Medical Director by means of written information.

All eligible and subsequently contacted neurological departments with an acute care mandate (n = 5), all intensive care units (n = 28) and all neurological rehabilitation clinics (n = 5) in Styria agreed to participate as study centres. The relevant department and clinic heads were then asked to nominate two doctors from their respective departments as contact persons, for example to ensure good continuity in the study process even during holiday periods. The contact persons were then centrally recorded by the study director using their names, telephone numbers and email addresses, and all study documents were sent to them. To ensure the study was not forgotten, all contact persons were subsequently contacted monthly by the study director via email and reminded of the key points of the study.

The respective interim analysis was also presented to encourage continued participation.

All contact persons received the study protocol, the ethics committee approval, the diagnostic criteria for apallic syndrome and the minimally conscious state in the ' ' (German translation and original publication), a consent form for guardians (see Ethics), the consent form for patients who may subsequently become capable of giving consent (see Ethics), and the contact details of the principal investigator.

All patients potentially eligible for inclusion in the study were reported to the principal investigator by the respective contact persons. For all wards not under neurological management, a neurological consultation was requested beforehand. All patients receiving analgesic sedation or mechanical ventilation, in whom the development of apallic syndrome could not be ruled out due to the acute event and the course of the illness, were also to be reported. The examination by the principal investigator was only carried out after the relevant sedation had ceased. The same applied to patients with high-grade febrile infections and other conditions complicating diagnosis, such as pronounced autonomic imbalances. The study centres are listed in the following table.

Table 6

Study centres

Hartberg Regional Hospital; Department of Anaesthesiology and Intensive

Care Medicine
Hartberg Regional Hospital; Internal Medicine Intensive Care Unit
Sigmund Freud Provincial Psychiatric Hospital; Intensive Care Unit and B-Rehab
Graz Trauma Centre; Intensive Care Unit
Voitsberg Regional Hospital; Intensive Care Unit
Leoben Regional Hospital; Intensive Care Unit
Deutschlandsberg Regional Hospital; Internal Medicine Intensive Care Unit
Deutschlandsberg Regional Hospital; Anaesthesiology
Tobelbad Rehabilitation Clinic
Kapfenberg Neurological Therapy Centre; B-Rehab
Kalwang Accident and Emergency Hospital; Intensive Care Unit
Wagna Regional Hospital; Intensive Care Unit
Bruck Regional Hospital; Intensive Care Unit
Lassnitzhöhe Rehabilitation Clinic
Judenburg Regional Hospital; Intensive Care Unit
Knittelfeld Regional Hospital; Intensive Care Unit
Hörgas-Enzenbach Regional Hospital; Intensive Care Unit
LKH West; Internal Medicine Intensive Care Unit
LKH West; Anaesthesiology
Maria Theresienklinik Radkersburg (Rehabilitation Clinic)
Fürstenfeld Regional Hospital; Intensive Care Unit
Feldbach Regional Hospital; Intensive Care Unit
Stolzalpe Regional Hospital; Intensive Care Unit
Schladming Hospital; Intensive Care Unit
Marienkrankenhaus Vorau; Intensive Care Unit
Rottenmann / Bad Aussee Hospital Group
Graz Regional Hospital; Medical Intensive Care Unit
Graz Regional Hospital; ICU 1 / Cardiac Transplant Intensive Care Unit
Graz Regional Hospital; ICU 2 / Anaesthesia Intensive Care Unit
Graz Regional Hospital; ICU 3 / Aseptic Intensive Care Unit
Graz Regional Hospital; ICU 4 / Septic Intensive Care Unit
Graz University Hospital; University Clinic for Surgery; Intensive Care Unit
Graz University Hospital; Neurosurgery Intensive Care Unit
Graz General Hospital; Neurology Intensive Care Unit
Hospital of the Brothers of Mercy, Graz; Intensive Care Unit
Mürzzuschlag General Hospital; Intensive Care Unit
Judendorf-Straßengel Rehabilitation Clinic
Hospital of the Sisters of St. Elizabeth; Intensive Care Unit

8.5 Inclusion and exclusion criteria

The inclusion and exclusion criteria listed below applied to the registration of potential study participants, although we also requested the registration of patients who might meet the criteria for a minimally conscious state. This was intended to ensure that, even in the event of misdiagnoses at the site, as complete a record as possible of individuals with apallic syndrome was obtained. Based on the research question of the Master's thesis, the criteria shown in Table 7 were established for the diagnosis of apallic syndrome and for inclusion in the study.

Table 7

Inclusion and exclusion criteria

Inclusion criteria: - Age 18 years or older - Main residence in Styria - Patients who, following a relevant acute event and subsequent comatose state, meet the diagnostic criteria of the 'Multi-Society Task Force on PVS' (1994). That is, all patients who awaken from a coma, open their eyes intermittently, but do not meet the required diagnostic criteria for 'minimally conscious state' according to Giacino (2002)
Exclusion criteria: - Progressive degenerative disease as the cause - ventilated or analgesically sedated patients (the examination was carried out at a as late as possible) - febrile infections or clinically manifest vegetative derailments (examination was carried out at the earliest possible later date)

8.6 Diagnosis and data collection

All diagnoses were made directly at the patient's bedside in the respective facility by the principal investigator. The principal investigator is a specialist in neurology with many years of experience in this field. In addition to the neurological examination, he took into account all previously available test results in his assessment of the patient's clinical condition. No additional tests were carried out solely for the purposes of the study.

8.6.1 *Clinical neurological examination*

The examination of the patients was carried out as accurately as possible, but no earlier than 4 weeks after the acute event. As already mentioned, a prerequisite for this was that there were no factors influencing the diagnosis, such as high fever or heavy sedation. Prior to the actual examination, a discussion took place with the attending doctor and the nursing staff and, where possible, with the patient's relatives.

In addition, the patient's medical records were reviewed. All of this was intended to ensure that signs of remission, which may have been subtle and intermittent during the course of the illness, could also be taken into account for the examination and diagnosis. The assessment of neurological status took into account the diagnostic criteria of the 'Multi-Society Task Force on PVS' (1994) as well as findings relevant to the differential diagnosis of the 'minimally conscious state'. The German version of these documents, translated by the study director, is included in the appendix.

8.6.2 *"Coma Recovery Scale Revised"*

In addition to the clinical neurological examination, the study director applied the "Coma Recovery Scale Revised" (CRS-R) – a scale frequently used in scientific research and well-validated – for an extended assessment, particularly with regard to the differential diagnosis of the "minimally conscious state" (Giacino et al. 2004).

In a paper by the "American Congress of Rehabilitation Medicine" (Seel et al. 2010), this scale was compared with numerous other scales in the assessment of patients with impaired consciousness. The comparison scales were the 'Sensory Stimulation Assessment Measure' (SSAM), the 'Wessex Head Injury Matrix' (WHIM), the 'Western Neuro Sensory Stimulation Profile' (WNSSP), the 'Sensory Modality Assessment Technique' (SMART), the 'Disorders of Consciousness Scale' (DOCS), the 'Coma/Near-Coma Scale' (CNC), the 'Full Outline of UnResponsiveness Score' (FOUR) and the 'Comprehensive Levels of Consciousness Scale' (CLOCS). This comparison showed that the CRS-R used is very well suited to distinguishing the minimally conscious state from the state of apallic syndrome. Furthermore, it proved effective due to its good practicality and relatively low time requirement. Extracts from the CRS-R manual are reproduced in German translation in the appendix.

8.6.3 *Collection of additional data*

In addition to determining whether reported patients met the clinical criteria for apallic syndrome or not, further data were collected. This included the age, gender and aetiology of the study patients. Of particular interest here was the question of whether the decline in traumatic causes reported in the literature would also be confirmed in this study. The duration of primary care, as well as the form and duration of subsequent care, were also recorded. Together with the recorded number of new cases, this data is intended to assist with future bed planning and the further optimisation of the care structure.

8.7 Ethics

Severely ill patients with no or severely impaired consciousness and an inability to communicate their own wishes and needs

must be given special protection from an ethical perspective.

The study proposal submitted to the Ethics Committee of the Medical University Hospital of Graz sought to take all these aspects into account and comprised the following documents: ethics application, study protocol, consent form for legal guardians, consent form for patients capable of giving retrospective consent. Medical supervision: The patient examination by the principal investigator was always carried out under the supervision of the care team.

Data confidentiality: The data collected during this study were treated as strictly confidential. For any potential publications, we undertook to publish all data only in anonymised form. To this end, patients were assigned a sequential two-digit numerical code.

CHAPTER 9

Incidence survey results

During the study period, a total of 39 patients with suspected full-blown apallic syndrome or a minimally conscious state were reported by the 38 study centres. Reports were made partly by telephone and partly by email, with the principal investigator always following up with a telephone call to the attending physician.

The primary suspected diagnosis was based on the precise diagnostic criteria for apallic syndrome and the minimally conscious state, which were provided to each study centre in the original version and in German translation at the start of the study. An additional neurological consultation was carried out in every case and was already available in most cases at the time of patient reporting.

A total of 9 patients died within 4 weeks of the acute event and thus before the principal investigator's examination.

In the case of a further 5 patients, no examination for study inclusion was carried out either, as a clear exclusion criterion was communicated by telephone by the attending physician within the first 4 weeks. In 4 of these cases, this involved a noticeable clinical improvement with clear signs of a 'minimally conscious state', and in 1 case, a patient with a definitive diagnosis of locked-in syndrome. All 5 patients were reported very early (within the first week) following the acute event.

Consequently, 25 patients were examined in person by the principal investigator no earlier than 4 weeks after the acute event (minimum 30 days; average 35.2 days; standard deviation 4.5 days; maximum 50 days). None of the patients examined were on controlled ventilation, receiving muscle relaxants or clinically relevant sedation at the time of examination.

One patient with a high-grade febrile infection and clinically significant autonomic derailment had to be examined a second time. During the first examination, this patient showed no signs of minimal consciousness, although it was unclear to what extent the reported deterioration in general condition was to blame for this. A few days later, after the patient's general condition had stabilised, the attending physician reported that the patient was showing clear signs of conscious activity. During the second examination, approximately four weeks later, a minimally conscious state was finally diagnosed, and the patient was therefore not included in the study. A further five reported individuals were also classified as MCS during the initial examination and were therefore not included in the study.

It is particularly emphasised that, as part of all investigations, the medical history and care records were reviewed in detail, and the attending doctors and nursing staff present were specifically questioned about the course of the illness and any signs of remission.

Ultimately, 19 patients were diagnosed with full-blown apallic syndrome (vegetative state) and were included in the study.

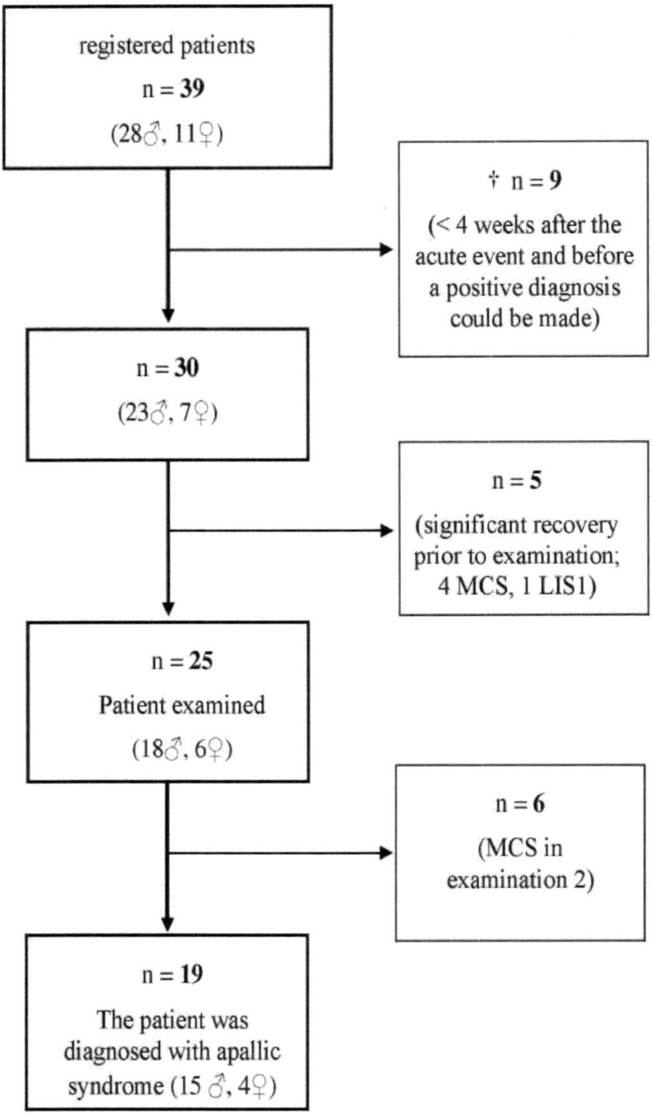

Figure 1: ***Overview of reported and included patients***

[1] LIS = Locked-in syndrome

[2] One patient was only classified as being in a 'minimally conscious state' (MCS) at the second examination.

The initial examination was not usable due to a febrile infection and vegetative dysregulation.

Table 8 provides an overview of the included patients. The following are listed , gender distribution, age, aetiology, CRS-R results and diagnoses.

Table 8

Overview of the included patients

Patient	Gender	Age	Aetiology	CRS-R	Diagnosis
1	m	18	Drugs	5	VS
2	w	64	Bolus response	4	VS
3	m	25	Traffic accident	5	VS
4	m	75	Myocardial infarction	2	VS
5	m	63	Aspiration	3	VS
6	m	58	Bolus administration	3	VS
7	w	59	SAB	2	VS
8	m	50	I	2	VS
9	m	78	Respiratory infection	3	VS
10	m	59	Traffic accident	6	VS
11	m	57	Myocardial infarction	2	VS
12	m	66	Myocardial infarction	5	VS
13	w	65	Ventricular fibrillation	2	VS
14	m	70	Myocardial infarction	5	VS
15	m	55	Ventricular fibrillation	3	VS
16	m	53	Myocardial infarction	3	VS
17	w	78	SAE	2	VS
18	m	57	SAE	6	VS
19	m	49	Traffic accident	4	VS

Abbreviations: SAH = subarachnoid haemorrhage; ICH = intracerebral haemorrhage; Respir. Insuff. = respiratory failure; PAE = pulmonary artery embolism; VS = vegetative state

9.1 Cumulative incidence in Styria

Based on the survey described above, 19 patients were diagnosed with full-blown apallic syndrome following an acute event during the study period (1 December 2011 – 30 November 2012). The total study population with their main residence in Styria and aged 18 years or older consisted of 1,010,164 individuals.

From this, the following incidence can be calculated:

$$\textbf{Cumulative incidence} = \frac{19 \times 100{,}000 \times 1}{1{,}010{,}164} = \textbf{1.88 / 100,000 / year}$$

Table 9 compares the incidence figures from various older studies with the data from this study. Some limitations in comparability arise from the specific features described in the notes.

Table 9

Comparison of incidence figures

Author	Incidence	Notes
Higashi (1977)	**2.47** per 100,000 per year or **0.82** per 100,000 per year [1]	with children; with degenerative diseases; inclusion ≥ 3 months after event
Sazbon (1992)	**0.4–0.5** per 100,000 per year	traumatic aetiology only
Beaumont (2005)	**0.5–2.5** per 100,000 per year	Diagnosis ≥ 6 months after the event
Von Wild (2007)	**0.5–2.0** per 100,000 per year	Summary; no primary epidemiological study
Pichler (2016)	**1.88** per 100,000 per year	≥ 18 years of age; no degenerative causes

[1] It is not clear from the publication whether the study period was 1 or 3 years (p. 25)

9.2 Age distribution in the present study

The youngest of our patients was 18 years old at the time of the acute event, the oldest 78 years old. The average age was 57.8 years (Figure 2).

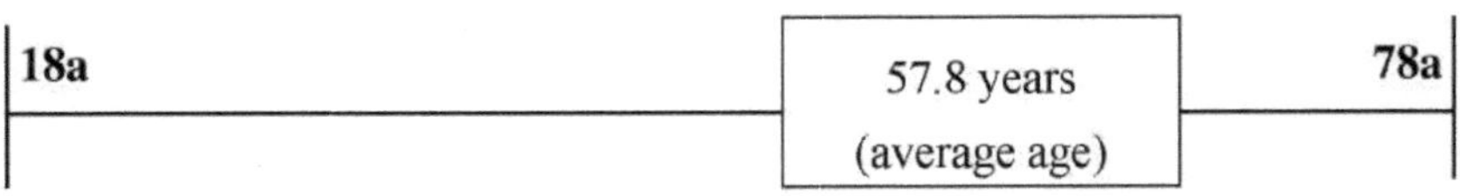

Figure 2: ***Age distribution of study patients***

(youngest patient; average age; oldest patient)

As the data on the total population can also be broken down by decade, we were able to calculate the incidence of apallic syndrome for specific age groups. Due to the very small numbers, we have grouped certain age ranges together for this purpose (Table 10).

Table 10: ***Incidence in different age groups***

Age	18–29 years	30–59 years	60 years and over
Population	186,205	525,029	298,930
Number	n = 2	n = 9	n = 8
Incidence	**1.07/100,000/year**	**1.71/100,000/year**	**2.68/100,000/year**
Gender	♂n = 2;♀ n = 0	♂n=8;♀ n=1	♂n = 5;♀ n = 3
CPR[1]	n = 1	n = 5	n = 7

[1] CPR = Cardiopulmonary resuscitation as the cause

Table 10 shows an age-related increase in the incidence of full-blown apallic syndrome (1.07/100,000/year for the 18–29 age group; 1.71/100,000/year for the 30–59 age group; 2.68/100,000/year for the age group 60 years and over).This differs significantly from the findings of Higashi (1977), in whose study the frequency of patients with apallic syndrome was distributed very evenly across the various age groups (0–20 years: n = 29 / 21–40 years: n = 27 / 41–60 years: n = 25 / >60 years: n = 29). It could be inferred from this that, at least in our part of the world, apallic syndrome is increasingly a condition of older age.

9.3 Gender distribution

The gender distribution is highly uneven (Figure 3). More than three-quarters of all participants were men (15 men, 4 women). Sazbon et al. (1990 & 1992) also reported in two studies that men were affected significantly more frequently (4:1 & 3.3:1). In the study by Higashi et al. (1977), 75 of the 110 patients included were men.

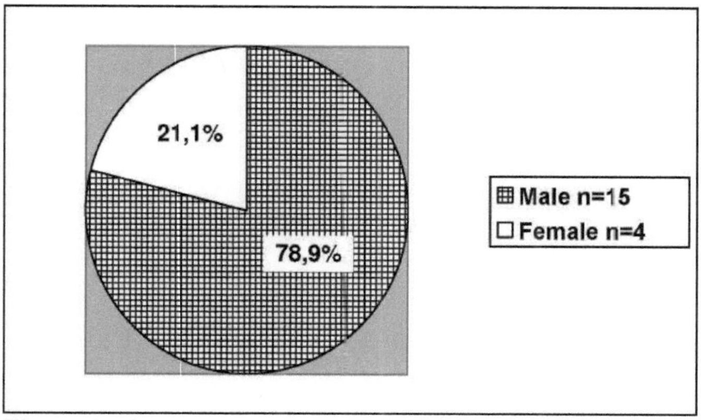

Figure 3: ***Gender distribution of the patients included***

1.4 Causes

With regard to the aetiological classification for the development of apallic syndrome, three groups can be identified in our study. By far the largest group comprised **hypoxic causes (n = 12)**. These were predominantly patients following cardiopulmonary resuscitation. The primary triggers were mainly cardiac events, but also bolus ingestion, aspiration and drug abuse (Figure 4). The other main groups were **traumatic brain injury (n = 3)** and intracranial **haemorrhage (n = 4)**.

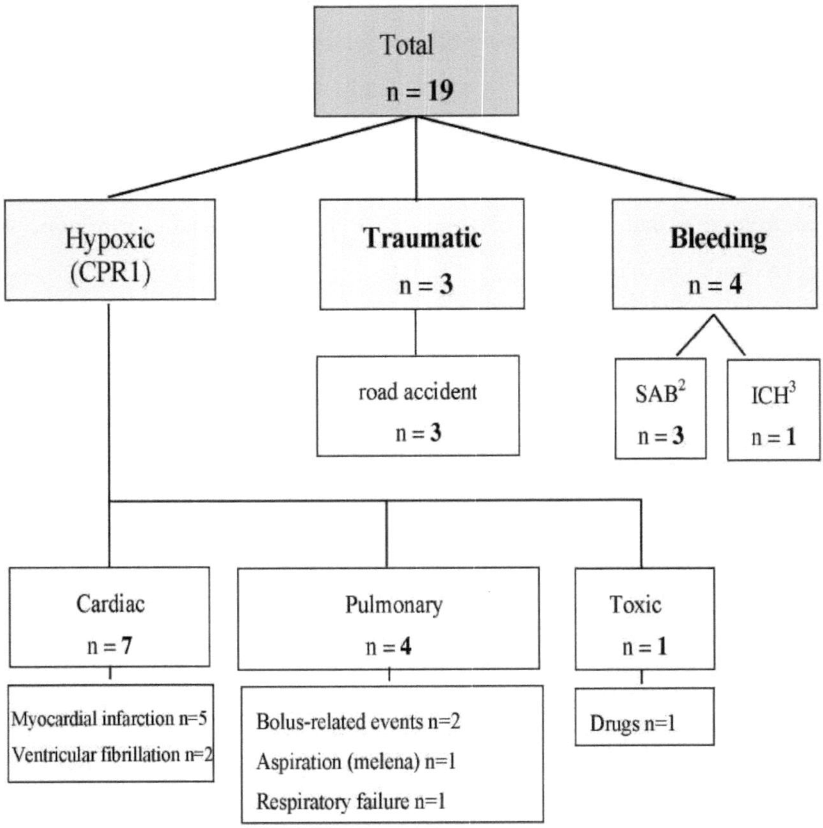

Figure 4: ***Aetiology of the study patients***

[1] Cardiopulmonary resuscitation; [2] Subarachnoid haemorrhage; [3] Intracerebral haematoma

The causes of illness in the reported but excluded individuals and the reasons for their exclusion are shown in Table 11.

Table 11

Overview of patients reported but not included

	Aetiology	Reason for exclusion
Hypoxia	CPR / myocardial infarction	MCS
	CPR / myocardial infarction	MCS
	CPR / myocardial infarction	MCS
	CPR / Myocardial infarction	deceased
	CPR / myocardial infarction	deceased
	CPR in the event of asystole	deceased
	CPR for ventricular fibrillation	deceased
	CPR following anaphylaxis	deceased
	Hypothermia	deceased
	Multiple myocardial infarction	MCS
Trauma	Road traffic accident	MCS
	Road traffic accident	MCS
	Road traffic accident	emerged MCS
	Traffic accident	emerged MCS
Haemorrhage	Brain stem haemorrhage	deceased
	brain stem haemorrhage	MCS
	Brain stem haemorrhage	Locked-in syndrome
	ICH associated with vascular malformation	deceased
	Aneurysm haemorrhage	MCS
Intoxication	Drugs	deceased

Abbreviations: CPR = cardiopulmonary resuscitation; MCS = minimally conscious state; ICH = intracerebral haemorrhage

CHAPTER 10

Epidemiology: Literature Review

The epidemiological figures on apallic syndrome available in the literature vary greatly. This is primarily due to differing diagnostic and inclusion criteria and varying times of diagnosis, which also suggests a high number of misdiagnoses. Overall, however, it is assumed that the number of patients with apallic syndrome is increasing in Europe (von Wild et al. 2007). Another reason for the rather unsatisfactory data situation is the fact that the prospective epidemiological studies required for these surveys are very time-consuming and, in most cases, also very costly.

10.1 Incidence

The known incidence figures for apallic syndrome vary greatly from country to country (see Table 14). This is understandable simply because there are significantly divergent rates of severe traumatic brain injury across different countries. For example, in the USA there are approximately 200 cases of severe traumatic brain injury per million inhabitants annually (Zasler et al. 1994). In England, the figure is estimated to be only about half of this number. How many of these patients ultimately develop apallic syndrome naturally also depends on the standard and availability of emergency medical services and the quality of intensive care, and thus also on economic factors.

Beaumont and Kenealy (2005) reported an incidence of 0.5–2.5 per 100,000 per year for patients who had been in a state of apallic syndrome for at least six months. Sazbon et al. (1992) provide high-quality data covering a 23-year period from Israel. Israel offers favourable conditions for epidemiological studies of apallic syndrome in that, one month after the acute event, all patients are transferred to a specialist centre (the 'Loewenstein Rehabilitation Hospital'). Thus, according t , a total of 580 patients with traumatic apallic syndrome (23.2 new cases per year) were documented between 1975 and 1998. From 1975 to 1983, there were an average of 16.3 patients per year, whilst the number rose significantly to 30 cases per year from 1983 to 1998. This results in an incidence of traumatic apallic syndrome in Israel of 0.4–0.5 per 100,000 per year. Non-traumatic cases were not included in this study.

Higashi (1977) also collected epidemiological data on apallic syndrome between 1973 and 1976 in collaboration with 269 hospitals in Japan. The study included all patients, regardless of the cause of the condition or their age, who had been in this clinical state for at least three months. Of the 269 institutions surveyed, 189 reported 193 potential patients, who were subsequently examined by the study team itself. Ultimately, a total of 110 patients were diagnosed as having apallic syndrome between 1973 and 1976. According to a sub-analysis, only 56 patients had a disease duration of less than 1 year (3 months – 1 year). However, the incidence was only recorded for one region with a population of approximately 1.5 million inhabitants, as comprehensive participation by healthcare facilities was only available there. For the 37 patients included in this population, this would result in an incidence of apallic syndrome in its full-blown form of 2.47 per 100,000. However, it is not clear from this study whether the study period for these 37 patients was also 3 years. This would then result in an incidence of 0.82 per 100,000 per year. A 'European Task Force' assumes an average incidence of 0.5–2 per 100,000 per year for apallic syndrome in its full-blown form (vegetative state), regardless of aetiology (von Wild et al. 2007). The authors also draw on individual data from France, Italy and Belgium. Some of these studies were written only in the respective national languages and could therefore not be investigated further here.

10.2 Prevalence

The prevalence of a condition also provides information about its chronicity and is therefore dependent on the incidence and the average survival time. Similar confounding factors and limitations to those encountered when collecting incidence figures also influence the collection of prevalence data. In addition, the nature and quality of long-term care, as well as differing country-specific legal frameworks on issues such as the discontinuation of artificial nutrition, play a significant role in this regard.

With regard to the 'average survival time' for persistent vegetative state (PVS), which is a key factor in calculating prevalence, the 'MultiSociety Task Force on PVS' (1994) reports a survival time of 2 to 5 years for patients who have survived for one month, and an average survival time of 10.5 years for patients who have survived the first year following the onset of the condition. This results in an estimate of 10,000–25,000 affected individuals in the USA, corresponding to a prevalence of 4–10 per 100,000 (The Multi-Society Task Force on PVS, 1994). In a more recent report for the USA, Jennett (2002) cites a prevalence among adults of between 40 and 168 per million inhabitants.

There are two studies on the prevalence of apallic syndrome in Austria. As of 28 November 2001, Stepan et al. (2004) surveyed the point prevalence of patients with full-blown apallic syndrome in Vienna. All 44 hospitals in Vienna and a total of 44 care facilities took part. Patient inclusion was based on a questionnaire used to record the patients' exact symptoms. As a plausibility check, the discharge diagnosis of 'apallic syndrome' from all hospitals in the Vienna Hospital Association (KAV) between 1996 and 2000 was compared with the study results. A total of 36 patients with apallic syndrome were identified at the study centres on that day. After excluding 4 patients who came from other countries, 32 patients were included. This resulted in a

point prevalence of 1.9 per 100,000. However, it should be noted that patients receiving care at home were not included in the data.

A further Austrian study investigating the prevalence of apallic syndrome was published by Donis and Kräftner (2011). The authors assessed the prevalence in Austrian long-term care facilities using telephone interviews. In the first step, the ward managers or medical directors of 889 facilities were contacted. 114 reported caring for patients with apallic syndrome or in a minimally conscious state. In the second step, the symptoms of the presumed patients in these 114 facilities were compared using a diagnostic checklist. The diagnostic criteria for the apallic syndrome (vegetative state) corresponded to those of the Multi-Society Task Force on PVS (1994), and the criteria for the minimally conscious state corresponded to those of Giacino et al. (2002). A total of 389 patients were identified (186 male, 203 female, average age 56.5 years). Of these, 269 met the criteria for apallic syndrome and 120 met the criteria for the minimally conscious state. This results in a prevalence of 3.36 per 100,000 for apallic syndrome and a prevalence of 1.5 per 100,000 for the minimally conscious state. In terms of aetiology, 22% were of traumatic origin, 27% were hypoxic in nature, 38% had occurred as a result of a stroke, cerebral haemorrhage or subarachnoid haemorrhage, and 13% had another aetiology (e.g. intoxication or infection). The average time elapsed since the acute event was between 2 and 5 years. Transfer from the acute care hospital to the long-term care facility usually took place after 3 to 12 months. A limitation of this study is that patients who were currently in an acute care hospital or a rehabilitation centre, as well as those receiving care at home, could not be included.

A similar study was conducted in the Netherlands by Lavrijsen et al. (2005). Patients presenting with the full clinical picture of apallic syndrome were surveyed across all care facilities. The study included 32 patients, resulting in a prevalence of just 0.2 per 100,000. This low figure may be explained by the prevailing legal situation in the Netherlands (active euthanasia) and by the moral and ethical approach to this patient group, which in principle differs from our own views. Whilst in countries where active euthanasia is permitted ( ), passive euthanasia through the withdrawal of nutrition and hydration is also discussed more extensively and the threshold for such action appears to be lower, in German-speaking countries the focus tends to be on discussions regarding the optimisation of patient care.

In their study covering the period 1979–1993, Engberg and Teasdale (2004) investigated the outcomes of patients following traumatic brain injury in Denmark. They found a point prevalence of 1.3 per million inhabitants for traumatic apallic syndrome five years after the event.

In their study on patients with full-blown apallic syndrome and the minimally conscious state in Northern Ireland, Wilson et al. (2002) reported a total prevalence of 23 per 1 million inhabitants.

In his review, Van Erb (2014) demonstrated a wide variation in the results of previous studies, ranging from 0.2 to 6.0 per 100,000. He attributes this to differences in the application of inclusion criteria and diagnostic procedures.

10.3 Aetiology

Etiologically, apallic syndrome can be divided into three main groups (Gerstenbrand, 1967). Acute severe brain damage, intoxication or chronic progressive cerebral processes are considered possible causes of this clinical picture (Table 12). The clinical symptoms are entirely independent of the cause. However, there are clear differences in terms of the prognosis and the course of the disease.

Table 12

Aetiology of apallic syndrome

Acute severe brain injury:		Trauma, hypoxia, encephalitis, etc.
Intoxication	- exogenous:	e.g. strychnine, mercury, manganese
	- endogenous:	e.g. hypoglycaemic, hepatic, uraemic
Degenerative	diseases:	Creutzfeldt-Jakob disease, Alzheimer's disease, Alzheimer's, Huntington's disease, etc.

The most common causes of acute severe brain damage are severe traumatic brain injuries, cerebral haemorrhages and, above all, cerebral hypoxia (e.g. following cardiopulmonary resuscitation, strangulation, being buried under rubble, near-drowning, stroke). Ultimately, however, any severe acute cerebral injury can cause apallic syndrome.

With regard to intoxications, it should be noted that a distinction must be made between exogenous and endogenous intoxications. An example of exogenous intoxication is drug overdose (Bruck & Gerstenbrand, 1967). Endogenous intoxications, such as uraemia, hyperglycaemia and hypoglycaemia, were described by Gerstenbrand et al. (1977), hyperthyroidism by Finkenstedt et al. (1974) and hepatitis by Binder (1981). Chronic intoxication can lead to apallic syndrome, either exogenously—for example, through mercury poisoning in the form of 'Minamata disease' (Gerstenbrand et al.

1977)—or endogenously through renal or hepatic failure.

Ultimately, chronic progressive cerebral diseases can also cause the symptoms of apallic syndrome. These severe degenerative diseases include, for example, various forms of dementia, Parkinson's disease, Huntington's disease or Creutzfeldt-Jakob disease. The full clinical picture of apallic syndrome represents, following a progressive process of brain degeneration, an absolute terminal stage with no possibility of regression.

The distribution of the various causes appears to change over time. Whilst Levy et al. (1981) stated in their publication that severe traumatic brain injury accounted for approximately 50% of cases of apallic syndrome, this proportion has declined significantly in later studies. For instance, von Wild et al. (2007) report that the frequency of traumatic brain injury as a cause is now only around one-third.

CHAPTER 11

Incidence Survey Discussion

Knowledge of the prevalence of a disease forms the basis of any serious engagement with this topic and also plays a decisive role in health economic planning. The data and study results on the incidence of apallic syndrome are inconsistent and, due to varying times of diagnosis and differing inclusion criteria (age, aetiology, etc.), are only comparable to a limited extent. Furthermore, the findings of the available studies can only be generalised to a limited extent, as there are sometimes significant differences between countries in the availability of emergency medical services and the number and quality of intensive care units. Social and legal differences between countries also play a significant role in this regard. To date, no published study has been conducted in Styria or Austria to determine the incidence of apallic syndrome, which is why the results of this study provide new and interesting data.

In the present study, an attempt was made to identify all acute patients with a final diagnosis of 'apallic syndrome' over a one-year study period. This diagnosis was recorded in adults aged 18 years and over, after excluding chronic degenerative diseases as the cause.

Insofar as it is comparable with other study results, the reported cumulative incidence of 1.88 per 100,000 per year lies at the upper end of the published data. Higashi et al. (1977) calculated an incidence of 2.47 per 100,000 per year in their work, but it must be noted that he also included children and patients with degenerative diseases as the cause. It is also not clearly stated whether the study period was 1 or 3 years. The incidence would possibly be reduced to 0.82 per 100,000 per year as a result (see 2.8.1 and Table 14). The results of Sazbon et al. (1992), on the other hand, are significantly lower th , although he only surveyed traumatic apallic syndrome (0.4–0.5 per 100,000 per year). In this regard, it should be noted that in the present study, the three traumatic patients included indicate an incidence of traumatic apallic syndrome in Styria of merely 0.3 per 100,000 per year. A European task force (von Wild et al. 2007) summarises the incidence across all age groups as 0.5–2.0 per 100,000 per year. The question of whether the incidence is generally on the rise cannot be answered, as the studies available differ too greatly in terms of methodology and inclusion and exclusion criteria.

In any case, a clear difference from earlier studies is evident with regard to the distribution of causes of the condition. Whilst older publications (Levy et al. 1981) the number of traumatic causes was still reported as approximately 50%, and Wild (2007) estimated this proportion at only about one-third, in the present study trauma was identified as the cause in only 3 out of 19 patients (incidence: 0.30 per 100,000 per year). Although precise epidemiological data on the severity and frequency of traumatic brain injuries are lacking for Austria (Oder, 2004), the analyses by Statistics Austria (www.statistik.at) do at least show a

decrease in road traffic accidents and casualties over the last 10 years, by around a fifth in each case (-19% and -21% respectively). Furthermore, the increasingly rapid availability of emergency medical care (e.g. via air ambulances) and the constantly improving standard of intensive care over the last few decades have led to a significantly better outcome following severe traumatic brain injury. Above all, the prevention of secondary damage plays a major role following traumatic events. The main causes of this secondary damage are arterial hypotension and hypoxaemia (Jeremitsky et al. 2003). In any case, monitoring intracranial pressure is crucial in treatment. The high prognostic value of intracranial pressure, particularly following traumatic brain injury, has been demonstrated repeatedly in studies (Hans et al. 1989; Jaggi et al. 1990). It is possible that, in the past, it was precisely these secondary injuries that were often partly responsible for the development of apallic syndrome following traumatic events. This, together with improvements in road safety over recent decades, appears to be responsible for the decline in the incidence of traumatic apallic syndrome.

However, in this study, the by far most common cause of apallic syndrome was cerebral hypoxia following cardiopulmonary resuscitation (see Figure 4). A similar trend was

also observed among the reported but excluded cases. Thanks to the aforementioned improvements in emergency and intensive care, an increasing number of patients are surviving cardiopulmonary resuscitation. Therapeutic hypothermia, which improves hypoxia tolerance, should be noted here as a scientifically validated intervention (Arrich et al. 2012). These appear to be the reasons why hypoxic causes of apallic syndrome are on the rise. The most common causes of hypoxic events were, in turn, cardiac events such as myocardial infarction and arrhythmias. These are primarily diseases of older age and are often associated with vascular risk factors. This likely explains the increasing number of hypoxic causes in older
age groups and the overall increase in incidence in older age groups (see Table 15). It is also noted that two reported patients had drug use as the cause (one patient was included, one patient died prior to the examination).

The uneven gender distribution was also striking (78.9% men). With the exception of one female patient, all individuals with hypoxic cardiac causes were male. Whether this uneven gender distribution is due to a different gender-specific cardiovascular risk profile, and whether women therefore suffer less frequently from cardiac arrests leading to apallic syndrome, cannot be answered by this study. The existing literature on this issue shows that the prevalence of female CHD is relatively low in the premenopausal period up to an average age of 51 years ( ) and only begins to align with that of men upon reaching the seventh decade of life (Shaw et al. 2006; Swahn, 1998). When breaking down the sexes into age subgroups, this study reveals a concentration of female cases in the older age group (see Table 15).

CHAPTER 12

Care structures in Austria

An optimised care pathway from the time of the acute event through to long-term care is crucial for the course of the disease and for the prevention of secondary and tertiary complications. Patients with apallic syndrome must receive continuous neurological care and be assessed regularly. Only in this way can misdiagnoses be avoided and the progression from apallic syndrome be recognised in good time. General treatment principles for patients with apallic syndrome are presented in Table 13.

Table 13

General treatment principles
- Regular neurological consultations, starting in intensive care units
- Timely detection of complications (e.g. increased intracranial pressure)
- Commencement of rehabilitation as soon as possible
- Formation of a multidisciplinary team (doctor, therapist, nursing staff)
- Development of an individualised neurorehabilitation programme
- Regular team meetings
- Regular neurological assessment

Key features in the management of this patient group include frequent recurrent infections in the urogenital tract and respiratory tract, as well as, in some cases, pronounced autonomic dysfunction. Nutrition and fluid intake are usually provided via a PEG tube. Many patients survive only with the aid of a tracheostomy tube or require ventricular shunt systems for adequate cerebrospinal fluid drainage and to regulate intracranial pressure. Occasionally, intrathecal pump systems are also implanted to administer antispastic agents. Complications and sudden deteriorations are possible at any time. This may, under certain circumstances, necessitate intensive care measures. In such cases, assessment by experienced doctors is particularly important, as 'maximum therapy' is often not effective and serious decisions—such as whether to reduce treatment— —must be made. A further distinctive feature of

care is the fact that patients are unable to communicate, and particular attention must be paid to early signs of remission. If signs of minimal consciousness appear, technical aids such as eye-tracking devices can also be used to facilitate potential communication.

12.1 Intensive care units

Intensive care serves, on the one hand, to stabilise vital signs and, on the other, to determine the cause (if unknown), to closely monitor the patient's progress and to plan further care. Above all, secondary ischaemic brain damage must be prevented through appropriate treatment. This is achieved through all measures proposed by the 'Austrian Resuscitation Council' in accordance with the 'European Resuscitation Council'. The view that, following severe traumatic brain injury, secondary hypoxic damage in particular can contribute to or even cause apallic syndrome is well-founded. No studies are available to clarify this issue. The utmost importance must therefore be placed on the development of neurologically and neurosurgically oriented intensive care medicine. In particular, intensive care physicians must be trained to the highest possible standard in the management of intracranial pressure, impaired cerebral perfusion pressure, the measurement of brain tissue oxygenation and the detection of metabolic crises. In non-neurologically managed intensive care units, close collaboration with a neurological consultant is of the utmost importance. In addition to clarifying the diagnosis, the clinical course must be recorded from the initial and transitional stages through to the full-blown apallic syndrome. However, the analgosedation frequently required makes this only partially possible.In patients with a poor prognosis, it may be possible to forgo maximum therapy in the event of additional severe complications (severe infections, haemorrhages, etc.). This decision should primarily be discussed within the interdisciplinary treatment team and must ultimately be determined by an ethics committee. For other affected patients, rehabilitation measures should begin whilst they are still in the intensive care unit. In principle, following successful stabilisation in intensive care, every patient with severe e brain damage should receive further care in a department offering early neurological rehabilitation. Transfer to suitable facilities should take place as soon as possible. Transfer directly from intensive care units to care homes or to home care, without a prior attempt at rehabilitation, is not justifiable. In exceptional cases where there is an acute shortage of beds in appropriate rehabilitation facilities, transfer to a specialised long-term care facility (known as a ‘vegetative state unit’ or ‘apallic care unit’) is possible. Should the regular neurological evaluations, which are mandatory here too, reveal signs of remission, transfer to a department for early neurological rehabilitation must be carried out as soon as possible.

12.2 Early neurological rehabilitation

Generally speaking, early neurological rehabilitation can be carried out in three differently structured organisational forms:

a) affiliated with a neuro-intensive care unit

b) integrated into an acute neurology ward

c) as an independent rehabilitation facility

The graduated options for neurorehabilitation in Austria are presented in a phased model.

Whilst vital functions are the primary focus in phases A and B, it is in the overlapping phases B, C and D that activities of daily living are relearned. The rehabilitation phases relevant to the various stages of remission for apallic syndrome are mostly phases A, B and C (Table 14).

Table 14
Phase model of neurorehabilitation in Austria

Phase A	Any acute neurological condition or acute deterioration of a chronic condition should be classified as Phase A during the first few days of treatment, as a significant level of diagnostic and acute therapeutic measures, including intensive care where necessary, is required.
Phase B	The patient experiences intermittent disturbances of consciousness and is unable to cooperate, or can do so only to a very limited extent. With regard to activities of daily living, they are completely or largely dependent on others. They do not require continuous ventilation; complications and emergency situations are frequent and

	may necessitate intensive care interventions, including temporary ventilation, at any time.
Phase C	The patient is alert, at least partially oriented, and is able to participate in therapeutic measures for three hours spread throughout the day.

Excerpt from: http://www.neuroreha.at/Phasenmodell.html

Patients with the full clinical picture of apallic syndrome meet all the criteria for Phase A in the acute phase and, subsequently, the criteria for neurological rehabilitation Phase B on a permanent basis, which is characterised as follows. Those affected have impaired consciousness, at least intermittently, and are unable to cooperate. Complications and emergency-like deteriorations may necessitate intensive care interventions, including temporary ventilation, at any time. In the event of a positive course of remission, where the patient's attention and cooperation are at least partially present and they are able to actively participate in therapies for several hours a day, transfer to a Phase C rehabilitation unit should be carried out. An individual rehabilitation programme must be drawn up for each patient. Precise, regular neurological examinations and discussions within the interdisciplinary team lead to the formulation of a prognosis and the continuous adaptation of the treatment programme. Special interventions, such as the implantation of baclofen pumps ( ), the use of botulinum toxin, surgery for ossifications or tendon lengthening in cases of contractures, should be considered where appropriate. When deciding to terminate rehabilitation treatment, the patient should be transferred to a so-called coma ward or, at the request of the guardian, arrangements should be made for transfer to a care home or home care. Transfer is appropriate if, despite sufficiently long and intensive rehabilitation efforts in Phase B, no improvement or no further trend towards improvement is apparent. For patients with a hypoxic cause, a rehabilitation trial of at least one month must be included in this assessment. In cases of traumatic aetiology, a longer period is advisable due to the generally better prognosis.

12.3 Long-term care

Patients with apallic syndrome constitute a group for whom specialised expertise in neurology, medicine and nursing is required, even in long-term care. In principle, care provision is designed to be long-term or is necessary as such, although the intensity of the measures may vary on an individual basis depending on various prognostic factors and the patients' needs. It has proved sensible to offer a tiered range of services in the long-term care sector as well. In Styria, long-term care for people is often provided in specialised facilities. The question of whether a patient is placed in a specialised coma care unit, a nursing home or receives home care depends, on the one hand, on the availability of beds in so-called coma care units, but is ultimately the responsibility of the patient's guardian.

12.3.1 Comatose wards

For some patients with severe damage to the central nervous system, significant long-term consequences of the condition persist despite adequate treatment in intensive care and subsequent neurorehabilitation. For these individuals, who can no longer live independently, intensive medical and therapeutic measures provided by an interdisciplinary team are necessary in addition to the care that is the primary focus . Therefore, to ensure a continuous chain of care, inpatient facilities must be established for all those affected who, despite every effort, remain in this condition indefinitely. These facilities must meet appropriate quality criteria that enable them to at least maintain, or even improve, the condition and remaining quality of life of those affected.

A milestone in quality assurance for such long-term care facilities (persistent vegetative state units) was achieved in Austria with the creation of an ÖNORM standard (ÖNORM K 1940:2011). This ÖNORM standard sets out the infrastructure, staffing requirements, processes and evaluation procedures for the care of patients with apallic syndrome, in order to meet the specific needs of this patient group. It serves as a guide for facilities and various professional groups dedicated to the care of this challenging patient group. However, it also acts as a decision-making aid for relatives, guardians and those responsible in the health and social care sectors, and serves as a basis for certification and assessment by the authorities. The tasks and objectives of long-term care facilities are outlined in Table 15.

Table 15

Tasks and objectives of long-term care facilities
- Safeguarding and monitoring the functional status achieved
- Identifying and avoiding factors that limit remission
- Improving communication and cooperation skills
- Continuation of sensory stimulation measures
- Maintaining the level of mobility achieved
- Monitoring and adjusting medical and pharmacological interventions
- Diagnosis, treatment and monitoring of medical complications, such as seizure disorders, autonomic dysfunction, tracheostomy tube management, recurrent respiratory and urogenital infections, vomiting, diarrhoea, dysphagia, aspiration, and food and fluid intake (possibly via PEG)
- Assessments to identify potential for rehabilitation
- Integration, support and training of relatives

Due to the varying needs of patients and in view of financial feasibility, care for patients in a persistent vegetative state has been divided into two phases in this ÖNORM:

Phase 1: Long-term neurological rehabilitation and supportive care (NLRF).

The aim of Phase 1 NLRF is to further improve the patient's condition and support them through additional rehabilitative measures. Patients should be admitted directly from rehabilitation facilities and, as already mentioned, only in exceptional cases directly from intensive care units or acute care hospitals. Prior to admission, a written assessment or an on-site examination of the patient must be carried out. The facility must be located near an acute hospital to ensure rapid access to diagnostic, therapeutic, acute medical or intensive care measures, with the hospital being reachable within 20 minutes. This ÖNORM standard also sets out the requirements for staff and the necessary staffing ratios (Table 16).

Table 16

Staff-to-patient ratios in long-term care facilities

	Phase 1 (NLRF)[a]	Phase 2 (NLBF)[b]
Doctor	1:20	1:20
Nursing	1.25:1	1:1
Physiotherapy	1:8	1:24
Occupational therapy	1:16	1:32
Speech therapy	1:32	1:96

From ÖNORM K 1940 (Structures for the long-term care of patients in a persistent vegetative state)

a NLRF = Long-term neurological rehabilitation and supportive care for people in a persistent vegetative state

b NLBF = Long-term neurological treatment and supportive care for people in a persistent vegetative state

Entry into the second phase of care is not defined by fixed time periods, but is based on the evaluation results of the interdisciplinary team experienced in caring for this patient group and on established scoring methods.

<u>Phase 2:</u> Long-term neurological treatment and supportive care for people in a persistent vegetative state (NLBF).

The aim of Phase 2 (NLBF) is to maintain the patient's condition through predominantly nursing care, but also therapeutic and medical measures. Should signs of remission appear, a transfer back from Phase 2 to Phase 1 or to a neurological rehabilitation facility is both possible and advisable.

Phase 2 wards should be regarded as long-term care facilities. Transfer to care homes close to the patient's home or to home care may be advantageous due to the proximity to the family environment and takes place with the consent or at the request of the guardian.

For both Phase 1 and Phase 2, process-oriented conditions must be established to ensure high-quality care. These include uniform care standards, standardised scoring systems, a standardised documentation system, regular team meetings, case conferences, supervision, as well as team development measures and structured in-service and training.

12.3.2 Nursing homes

Following stabilisation in intensive care and the completion of the rehabilitation phase, nursing homes are also available for the long-term care of people in a persistent vegetative state. In this context, it should be noted that whilst the intensity of medical care and therapeutic requirements decrease in the long-term care sector, the level of nursing care required remains consistently high. Therefore, appropriate requirements must also be set for nursing homes caring for patients in a persistent vegetative state, particularly in the area of nursing care. These relate both to the staff-to-patient ratio and to the qualifications of the nursing staff. Furthermore, therapeutic measures to maintain function must be implemented, and neurological monitoring, at least in the form of a neurological consultation service, must be required. In summary, the ÖNROM guidelines (Phase 2 NLBF) should also be required for nursing homes.

12.3.3 Home care

To ensure continued care at home, the needs of patients due for discharge and of the relatives requiring support should be identified prior to discharge. Appropriate structural and quality criteria for home care must be developed. Discharge management should be viewed against the backdrop of ensuring that patients receive adequate care following a prolonged inpatient stay, whilst minimising the burden on their relatives.

Timely discharge is made possible by 'early discharge management', as preparations made during the inpatient stay for further care at home ensure the greatest possible safety and thereby encourage the willingness to take the patient home. Training sessions for family carers delivered by nursing staff and therapists have proven just as effective as close collaboration with the relevant GPs. This improves the quality of discharge and should be offered by all institutions.

The following points should be considered for discharge to the home:

- Ensuring professional follow-up care is in place before discharge
- If necessary, organising a mobile team of therapists with flexible availability
- Drawing up an individual outpatient rehabilitation programme
- Development and dissemination of standards for patient management
- Maintaining contact with the discharging facility to provide assistance in difficult situations and to answer questions from relatives.

CHAPTER 13

Care pathway of the study patients

A further aim of this study was to map the care pathway of those affected. These data are also important for further optimising care planning and could be incorporated into the development of the 'Regional Health Structure Plan' (RSG) in the future.

With regard to the existing care structures in Styria, it was found that just over half (8 out of 15) of the patients who were discharged from an intensive care unit were admitted to a department for early neurological rehabilitation. This lasted an average of 65 days, which, given the high proportion of hypoxic brain injuries, appears sufficient for a therapeutic trial and a prognostic assessment of the overall situation. The objective desired by the professional associations: "Every patient with severe brain injury should have access to a rehabilitation trial", has not been achieved. Of the 8 individuals who received early neurological rehabilitation, all 5 registered at the coma unit were admitted (1 patient died prior to admission and 2 were cared for at home at the request of their relatives). A further 6 patients were admitted directly to the coma unit from intensive care units and 1 patient from the inpatient ward of an acute care hospital. Although this generally contradicts the aim of a tiered rehabilitative care system, it ultimately reflects the fact that waiting times for admission to early neurological rehabilitation units are too long for patients with apallic syndrome, or that there is a greater need for beds in this area. During the study period, the coma unit at the Albert Schweitzer Clinic in Graz was able to admit all registered patients for inpatient care.

Despite discussions with members of the care team and a review of the patient's medical records, the clinical assessment and evaluation carried out using the CRS-R ultimately provides only a snapshot of the patient's condition at that particular moment. However, it is to be expected that, through the continued care of most surviving patients in the coma unit at the Albert Schweitzer Clinic in Graz and through further evaluation as part of the 1-year follow-up, additional data can be generated to confirm the results.

The question of whether all those affected were actually reported cannot, ultimately, be answered with absolute certainty. In any case, there are many indications to suggest this. For instance, the very even distribution of patient reports throughout the entire study year and the large number of different reporting centres suggest good and active participation by the collaborating partners and thus a high level of representativeness of the reports. The large number of reported individuals (n = 39) compared to the number of included individuals (n = 19) also suggests motivated participation by the collaborating partners and rules out the possibility of selection bias.

The fact that all intensive care units, all neurological departments and all neurological rehabilitation clinics in Styria took part in this incidence survey further speaks in favour of the study's high quality. Other positive aspects include the relatively long one-year study period, the precise and up-to-date data set on the population, the precise diagnostic criteria, the consistent timing of examinations, and the consideration of factors that could bias the diagnosis, such as fever or autonomic dysfunction. As all patients were examined by the same neurologist with expertise in this field, the issue of inter-rater variability does not arise.

In summary, this study found an incidence of apallic syndrome of 1.88 per 100,000 per year, which is in the upper normal range compared to the existing literature. When considered for Austria as a whole and for countries with similar conditions and a similar standard of healthcare, the results of this study can certainly also be used as a 'benchmark' for estimating the incidence in those regions. A tiered rehabilitative care system for patients appears to be well established in Styria, although there is a need for additional beds for early neurological rehabilitation of this patient group. No conclusions can be drawn regarding the prevalence and care situation of infants, children and adolescents. Looking ahead, it is worth noting that the second part of this epidemiological study, which focuses on the '1-year follow-up' of the study patients included, has already begun. This will yield further information on the current care situation. In particular, key figures such as the incidence of infections or the number of readmissions to an acute care hospital can be collected. To confirm the study results and identify trends over time, this study should be repeated in a few years' time and, if possible, conducted in a comparable format in other Austrian federal states as well. Through collaboration between the various healthcare facilities, this would certainly be feasible under the coordination of the neurological professional association. A further objective would be to extend the incidence survey to include the clinical conditions 'minimally conscious state' and 'locked-in syndrome'.

As expected, every patient with a final diagnosis of apallic syndrome was initially treated in an **intensive care unit**. The average length of stay was 22.7 days (minimum 10 days; maximum 48 days). Four of these 19 patients died in the intensive care units where they were being treated. Of the 15 survivors, 8 were admitted to **early neurological rehabilitation** (Phase B). Six patients were transferred directly from the intensive care units to the **coma unit** at the Albert Schweitzer Clinic in Graz. Another patient was cared for on a general ward in the acute hospital **for** 11 days prior to admission to the **coma unit**. All 8 patients who underwent early neurological rehabilitation were treated in the Neurology Department of the Sigmund Freud Provincial Neurological Clinic (LSF). The average duration of rehabilitation was 65 days (minimum 16 days [this patient died]; maximum 84 days). Five patients received further care on the coma ward of the Albert Schweitzer Clinic, and two patients were discharged directly from early rehabilitation to **home care** . In total, 12 of the 14 study patients who have survived to date were admitted to the coma ward. The average length of stay is not meaningful in this context, as at the time of evaluation for this master's thesis, the stay had not yet ended for many patients. It should be noted that one reported patient received acute treatment in another federal state and was only subsequently transferred to Styria for neurological rehabilitation. This demonstrates the value of all rehabilitation clinics participating in this study. However, this patient was ultimately not diagnosed as being in a state of apallic syndrome. Figures 5 and 6 illustrate the care pathway for the study patients included.

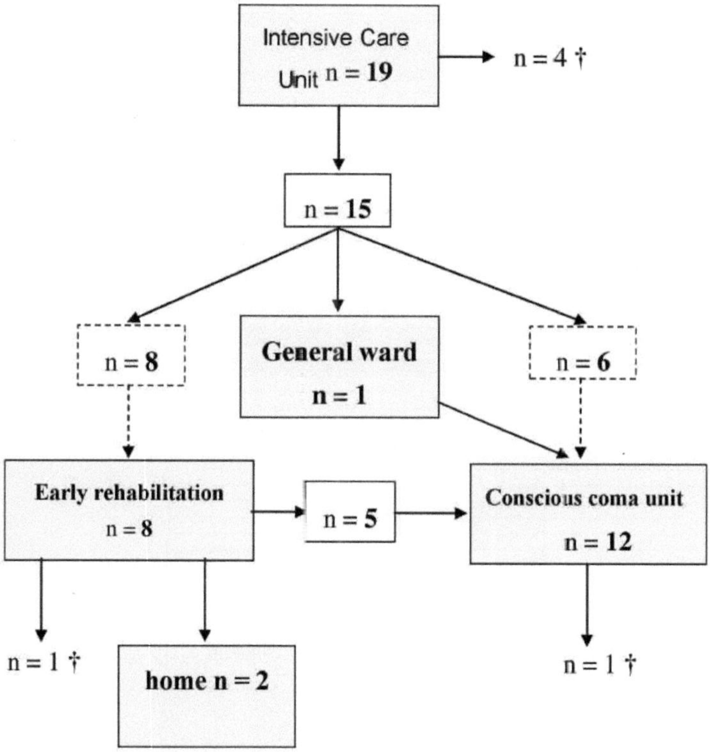

Figure 5: ***Illustration of patient care***

The second part of the study (1-year follow-up) has already begun, but no meaningful data are available yet. The main focus is on tracking and presenting the clinical courses of the 13 study participants who are currently still alive. The primary areas of interest are changes in the clinical course, the number of acute interventions required, and the form of ongoing care.

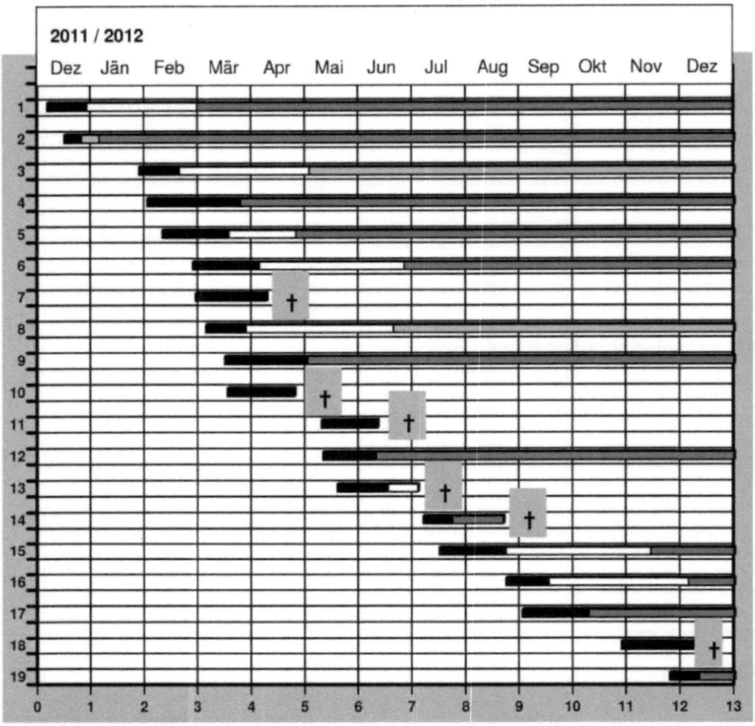

Figure 6: ***Care facilities and duration of care***

Intensive care unit B-Rehab Conscious coma unit At home

† = deceased

CHAPTER 14

Optimised 'Styria' model for the care of patients in a persistent vegetative state

14.1 Aspects of care quality

Since the partial funding of 20 persistent vegetative state beds by the Styrian Health Fund, annual admission figures had almost quintupled by 2015 (Figure 7). Given that the admission criteria take into account not only patients in a persistent vegetative state (PVS) but also those in the early stages of recovery (MCS) and with locked-in syndrome, the admission of 26 new patients in 2015 is consistent with the incidence of PVS. It is also a key objective of the Coma Unit to ensure that all patients receive appropriate follow-up care following the completion of acute treatment or early rehabilitation.

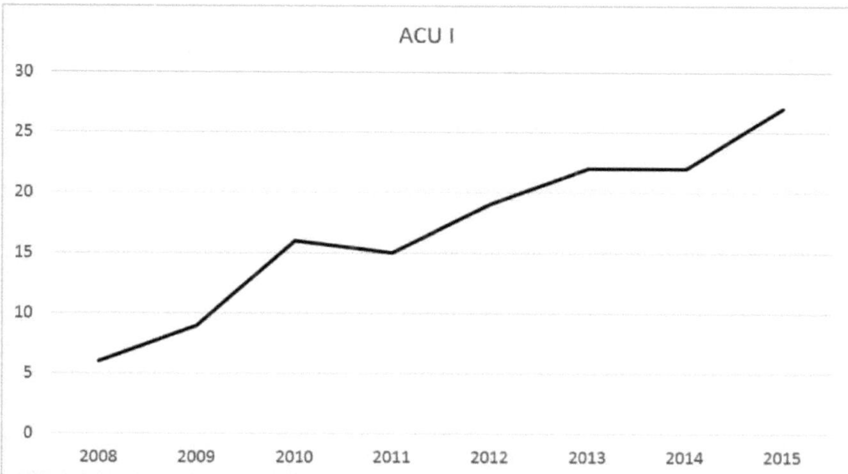

Figure 7: ***Trend in admission figures for the coma unit***

Trend in admission figures (including readmissions) to the coma unit, which is partially funded by the Health Fund.

Based on years of experience, this care unit has also increasingly established itself and proven its worth as **a triage ward** (Figure 8). In addition to relieving the pressure on the intensive care units of Styrian hospitals as quickly as possible ( ), the aim is to provide treatment tailored to patients' needs, comprising the following:

Stabilisation of the patient's general condition using non-intensive care measures and identification of potential for rehabilitation. This is ensured through continuous observation by a specialist neurologist and regular interdisciplinary assessments on the coma ward. Direct transfer from the intensive care units to a care home would largely deprive the patient of the chance of identifying a 'late improvement'.

Rehabilitation preparation: If a clear potential for recovery emerges at a later stage, patients may also be referred to the rehabilitation process at a later stage. To this end, close contact has been established with Styrian rehabilitation facilities in recent years. Readmission for the purpose of planning subsequent home care is possible and also advisable in individual cases.

Palliative care: For patients with extremely severe injuries and no prospect of stabilisation or improvement, palliative care involving a restriction of maximum treatment may be initiated, taking ethical considerations into account. This is done after informing and consulting the patient's legal representative or relatives. The patient's presumed wishes or those set out in writing, for example in the form of a living will, must in any case be taken into account.

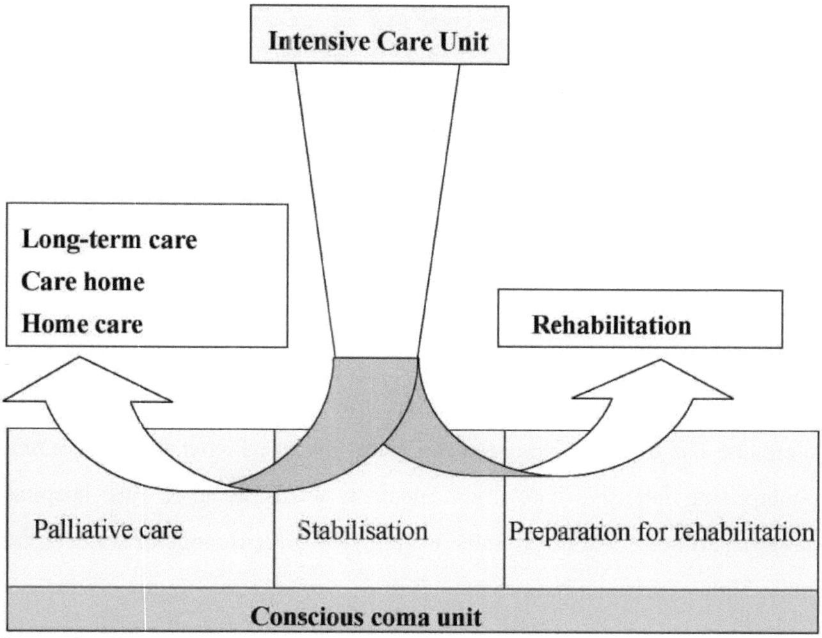

Figure 8: ***Triage function of a coma unit***

In order to transfer patients to a suitable care facility as quickly as possible and, above all, at the right time, with a view to ensuring optimal treatment quality, the following approach is considered appropriate in light of the current situation in Styria, from the perspective of the Coma Unit at the Albert Schweitzer Clinic Graz:

Maintaining the high profile of the coma unit's services to **ensure the best possible relief** for **intensive care units, neurological departments** and **rehabilitation facilities** through the rapid transfer of patients. This can be achieved through regular information letters, joint meetings or within the context of scientific work, such as the study described in this book. **Younger, working patients with a good prognosis** must be transferred primarily to a **rehabilitation facility**. **Older patients, particularly those with hypoxic causes and the associated poorer prognosis**, can be transferred **directly to a coma unit in the first instance** to ensure optimal quality of care in line with the triage function mentioned above. In line with the increasing age of those affected and the shift in the aetiology of coma demonstrated in our study, this recommendation will become even more important in the future.

If home care or transfer to a care home close to the patient's home is desired by the relatives or the patient's guardian, appropriate guidance and training must be provided. Continued outpatient medical care must be ensured by the responsible GP.

14.2 Economic aspects

Co-authors:
Hon. Prof. (FH) Dipl.-HTL-Ing. Mag. Dr. Gerd Hartinger MPH
Harald Fuchs, BSc

In addition to optimising the quality of care, this chapter also discusses health economic effects. The facilities along the care pathway for patients with severe brain damage, comprising intensive care units, inpatient wards in acute care hospitals, rehabilitation departments and coma units, have a very diverse range of services and, consequently, highly varied daily rates.

Daily rates in Styria 2015 (€)

Intensive care units (s)	1,157.54
General ward, Graz University Hospital	932.20
Mixed rate for other regional hospitals	674.80
Early rehabilitation, phase B	506.84
Conscious coma unit	325.40

Intensive care units are classified into three levels depending on the level of care required. For 2013, the weighted average level is 2.33. This corresponds to a daily rate of €1,157.54, calculated using the average Styrian LKF point value for 2015 (as full cost coverage).

These widely varying daily rates reflect the differences in the services provided (see Chapter 12). It is important, both for the quality of care and for the costs incurred, that patients are given access to appropriate services as quickly as possible and that the treatment pathway is tailored to the patient's potential for recovery. Consequently, provided it is medically indicated, transferring patients as quickly as possible to an appropriate but more cost-effective care unit leads to savings for the healthcare system.

The triage function of the coma ward also serves to facilitate the targeted secondary referral of patients to other care units (e.g. Phase B early neurological rehabilitation). The resulting overall reduction in primary referrals avoids a 'scattergun approach', without, however, preventing patients from having all rehabilitation options open to them should appropriate signs of remission appear.

These synergy effects have been made possible by years of experience and a care pathway that is extremely finely tuned with all healthcare facilities.

Figure 9 illustrates, by way of example, the patient pathways from the perspective of the coma unit in 2015. The advantages arising, in our view, from this model of 'Styrian coma care' are described below for each pathway.

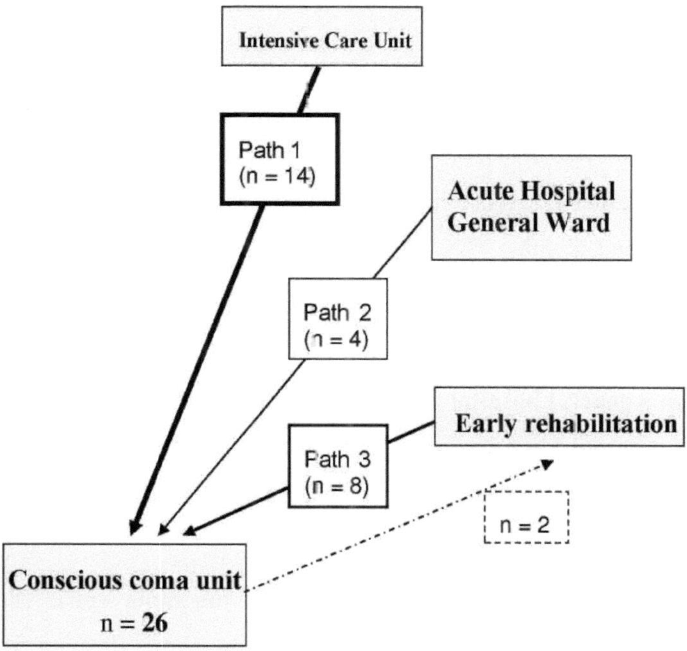

Figure 9: ***Care pathways 2015***

(n=26; 1 readmission was not included)

Path 1 (direct transfer from the intensive care unit to the coma care unit): In the interests of targeted early intervention, patients should be transferred from intensive care units to specialised treatment facilities as quickly as possible once intensive care measures have been completed. Not least due to limited bed capacity and for economic reasons, the **stay**

in intensive care units should be kept **as short as possible**. Rapid patient transfer is therefore of particular importance. Thanks to an internal process for patient assessment and transfer, any medically suitable patient with their main residence in Styria can be admitted swiftly to the coma care unit. This currently takes place on average 8 days after initial contact with the referring doctor. However, this should often not be regarded as the total waiting time, as at the time of initial registration, specific investigations may still be pending or intensive care interventions (such as weaning from ventilation) may not yet have been completed. The waiting time until neurological early rehabilitation (Phase B) is currently estimated at 2–3 weeks.

During 2015, only 2 patients from Pathway 1 showed corresponding improvements during regular evaluations on the coma ward, and these were also referred to early rehabilitation. However, for the majority of patients admitted directly from the intensive care unit, no corresponding rehabilitation potential was evident even over the course of further weeks and months. This means that the highly specialised early rehabilitation treatment places were used sparingly, and it underlines the importance of **the coma unit's triage function**.

Path 2 (Transfer from a general hospital ward to the coma ward): Transfers from the acute hospital ward as quickly as possible and targeted secondary referrals to rehabilitation facilities can also be regarded as significant opportunities for cost savings in Path 2.

Path 3 (Transfer from an early rehabilitation facility to the coma unit): The possibility of subsequent transfer to a coma unit facilitates discharge planning for rehabilitation facilities. This involves specialised follow-up care with a range of rehabilitation services, long-term care with medical supervision, or, in many cases, preparation for discharge to the patient's home.

Thanks to the tiered care model in the coma care units at the Albert Schweitzer Clinic in Graz, unnecessary costs can also be avoided in Pathway 3.

In summary, the tiered Styrian care model for patients in a persistent vegetative state represents a sensible approach to optimising care for patients with severe consciousness disorders. The coma ward primarily serves a triage function in this context. From a health economics perspective, the rapid transfers from the acute hospital sector (intensive care units) and the targeted secondary referrals to rehabilitation facilities are likely to have the greatest impact. The low number of readmissions to acute care hospitals (, e.g. in the case of relatively common infections of the respiratory and urinary tracts requiring treatment) represents a further synergy effect of a coma ward with a mandate for long-term care, as opposed to purely nursing care. This article has deliberately refrained from attempting a monetary evaluation of the described effects due to the still low absolute figures and the complexity of cost models.

REFERENCES

Adams, JH. Graham, DI. Murray, LS. & Scott, G. (1982). Diffuse axonal injury due to non-blunt head injury in humans: an analysis of 45 cases. Ann Neurol. 12(6):557-63.

Aichner, F., Gerstenbrand, F. & Poewe, W. (1982–1983). Primitive motor patterns and stereotyped movements. A comparison of findings in early childhood and in the apallic syndrome. Int J Neurol, 16–17:21–9.

Andrews, K. (1993). Recovery of patients after four months or more in the persistent vegetative state. BMJ, 12;306(6892):1597-600.

Andrews, K., Murphy, L., Munday, R. & Littlewood, C. (1996). Misdiagnosis of the vegetative state: retrospective study in a rehabilitation unit. BMJ, 6;313(7048):13-6.

Arrich, J., Holzer, M., Havel, C., Müllner, M. & Herkner, H. (2012). Hypothermia for neuroprotection in adults after cardiopulmonary resuscitation. Cochrane Database of Systematic Reviews, 12;9:CD004128.

Artner Dworzak, E. Secnik, P. Parrak, V. Puschendorf, B. Marosi, M. Muigg, A. Gerstenbrand, F. & Koller, A. (1993). Changes in muscular proteins during simulated microgravity. J Neurol Sci, 119(1):119-20.

Bates, D. (2005). The vegetative state and the Royal College of Physicians guidance. Neuropsychol Rehabil, 15(3-4):175-83.

Bauer, G., Gerstenbrand, F. & Aichner, F. (1983). Locked-in syndrome: pseudocoma following pons sections. Psychiatr Neurol Med Psychol, 29:139-45.

Bauer, G., Gerstenbrand, F. & Rumpl, E. (1979). Varieties of the locked-in syndrome. J Neurol, 221(2):77-91.

Beaumont, JG. & Kenealy, PM. (2005). Incidence and prevalence of the vegetative and minimally conscious states. Neuropsychol Rehabil, 15(3-4):184-9.

Binder, H. (1981). On the neuropsychiatric symptomatology of the so-called 'hepatic coma'. Wien Klin Wochenschr Suppl, 134:1-19.

Bruck, J. & Gerstenbrand, F. (1967). Functional decerebration presenting the picture of an apallic syndrome due to high-dose majeptil therapy. A contribution to the question of the mode of action and site of action of certain neuroleptics. Nervenarzt, 38(10):459-64.

Butler, A.B., Manger, P.R., Lindahl, B.I. & Arhem, P. (2005). Evolution of the neural basis of consciousness: a bird-mammal comparison. Bioessays 27, 923–936.

Childs, N.L., Mercer, W.N. & Childs, H.W. (1993). Accuracy of diagnosis of persistent vegetative state. Neurology, 43(8):1465-7.

Dehaene, S., Changeux, J.P., Naccache, L., Sackur, J. & Sergent, C. (2006). Conscious, preconscious and subliminal processing: a testable taxonomy. Trends Cogn Sci 10, 204–211.

Donis, J. & Kräftner, B. (2011). The prevalence of patients in a vegetative state and minimally conscious state in nursing homes in Austria. Brain Injury, 25(11): 1101-1107.

Engberg, AW. & Teasdale, TW. (2004). A population-based study of survival and discharge status among survivors of head injury. Acta Neurol Scand, 110(5):281-90.

Finkenstedt, G., Binder, H., Gerstenbrand, F., Kleinberger, G., Kotzaurek, R., Lesch, O., Mamoli, B., Pall, H., Pichler, M., Raberger, G. & Szeless, S. (1974). Unusual course of thyrotoxicosis masked as a neuropsychiatric disorder. Wien Klin Wochenschr, 6;86(16):476-80.

Formisano, R., Saltuari, L. & Gerstenbrand, F. (1995). Presence of Kluver-Bucy syndrome as a positive prognostic feature for the remission of traumatic prolonged disturbances of consciousness. Acta Neurol Scand, 91(1):54-7.

Gerstenbrand, F. (1967). The traumatic apallic syndrome. Vienna: Springer.

Gerstenbrand, F., Avenarius, H.J. & Preissler, H.P. (1977). The apallic syndrome in metabolic disorders of the brain. Monogr Gesamtgeb Psychiatry Ser, 14:29–36.

Gerstenbrand, F., Hamdi, T., Kothbauer, P., Rustam, H. & Al Badri, M. (1977). Apallic syndrome in chronic mercury poisoning. Eur Neurol, 15(5):249-56.

Gerstenbrand, F., Poewe, W., Aichner, F. & Saltuari, L. (1983). Klüver-Bucy syndrome in man: experiences with post-traumatic cases. Neurosci Biobehav Rev, 7(3):413-7.

Giacino, JT. Ashwal, S. Childs, N. Cranford, R. Jennett, B. Katz, DI. Kelly, JP. Rosenberg, JH. Whyte, J. Zafonte, RD. & Zasler, ND. (2002). The minimally conscious state: definition and diagnostic criteria. Neurology, 12;58(3):349-53.

Giacino, J., Kalmar, K. & Whyte, J. (2004). The JFK Coma Recovery Scale-Revised: Measurement--characteristics and diagnostic utility. Archives of Physical Medicine and Rehabilitation, 85(12):2020-2029.

Gill-Thwaites, H. (1997). The Sensory Modality Assessment Rehabilitation Technique: a tool for the assessment and treatment of patients with severe brain injury in a vegetative state. Brain Inj, 11(10):723-34.

Gill-Thwaites, H. & Munday, R. (2004). The Sensory Modality Assessment and Rehabilitation Technique (SMART): a valid and reliable assessment for patients in a vegetative state and minimally conscious state. Brain Inj, 18(12):1255-69.

Hans, P., Albert, A., Franssen, C. & Born, J. (1989). Improved outcome prediction based on CSF-extrapolated creatine kinase BB isoenzyme activity and other risk factors in severe head injury. J Neurosurg, 71:54-8.

Higashi, K., Hatano, M., Abiko, S., Ihara, K., Katayama, S., Wakuta, Y., Okamura, T. & Yamashita, T. (1981). Five-year follow-up study of patients with persistent vegetative state. J Neurol Neurosurg Psychiatry, 44(6):552-4.

Higashi, K., Sakata, Y., Hatano, M., Abiko, S., Ihara, K., Katayama, S., Wakuta, Y., Okamura, T., Ueda, H., Zenke, M. & Aoki, H. (1977). Epidemiological studies on patients with a persistent vegetative state. J Neurol Neurosurg Psychiatry, 40(9):876-85.

Jaggi, JL. Obrist, WD. Gennarelli, TA. & Langfitt, TW. (1990). Relationship of early cerebral blood flow and metabolism in acute head injury. J Neurosurg, 72:176-82.

Jellinger, K. (1968). On the neuropathology of coma and post-comatose encephalopathies. Wien Klin Wochenschr, J28;80(26):505-9.

Jellinger, K. (1977). Pathology and pathogenesis of apallic syndromes following closed head injuries. Monogr Gesamtgeb Psychiatr Psychiatry Ser, 14:88-103.

Jellinger, K. (1994). The brain of Karen Ann Quinlan. N Engl J Med, 17;331 (20):1378-9; author reply 1379-80.

Jellinger, K. (2009). Functional pathophysiology of consciousness. Neuropsychiatry, Vol. 23, No. 2, pp. 115–133.

Jellinger, K., Gerstenbrand, F. & Pateisky, K. (1963). The protracted form of post-traumatic encephalopathy. Clinical and morphological findings following severe closed craniocerebral trauma with long- -survival. Nervenarzt, 34:145–59.

Jennet, B. (2002a). The vegetative state. Medical facts, ethical and legal dilemmas. Cambridge University Press.

Jennett, B. (2002b). The vegetative state. J Neurol Neurosurg Psychiatry, 73(4):355-7.

Jennett, B., Cranford, R. & Zasler, N. (1997). A consensus statement on criteria for the persistent vegetative state is being developed. BMJ, 314(7094), 1621-2.

Jennett, B. & Plum, F. (1972). Persistent vegetative state after brain damage. A syndrome in search of a name. Lancet, 1(7753), 734-7.

Jeremitsky, E., Omert, L., Dunham, CM., & Rodriguez, A. (2003). Harbingers of poor outcome the day after severe brain injury: hypothermia, hypoxia, and hypoperfusion. J Trauma, 54: 312–19.

Kampfl, A., Schmutzhard, E., Franz, G., Pfausler, B., Haring, H.P., Ulmer, H., Felber, S., Golaszewski, S., & Aichner, F. (1998). Prediction of recovery from post-traumatic vegetative state with cerebral magnetic-resonance imaging. Lancet, 13;351 (9118):1763-7.

Kinney, HC. & Samuels, MA. (1994). Neuropathology of the persistent vegetative state. A review. J Neuropathol Exp Neurol, 53(6):548-58.

Kretschmer, E. (1940). The apallic syndrome. Z ges Neurol Psychiat, 169:576-579.

Laureys, S., Celesia, G. G., Cohadon, F., Lavrijsen, J., Leon-Carrion, J., Sannita, W. G., Sazbon, L., Schmutzhard, E., von Wild, K. R., Zeman, A. & Dolce, G. European Task Force on Disorders of Consciousness. (2010). Unresponsive wakefulness syndrome: a new name for the vegetative state or apallic syndrome. BMC, 1;8:68.

Lavrijsen, J. Van den Bosch, J S G. Koopmans, R. & Van Weel, C. (2005). Prevalence and characteristics of patients in a vegetative state in Dutch nursing homes. J Neurol Neurosurg Psychiatry, 76(10):1420-1424.

Lechinger, J., Chwala-Schlegel, N., Fellinger, R., Donis, J., Michitsch, G., Pichler, G., & Schabus, M. (2013). Mirroring of a simple motor behaviour in disorders of consciousness. Clin Neurophysiol, 124(1):27-34.

Lerner, DJ. & Kannel, WB. (1986). Patterns of coronary heart disease morbidity and mortality in the -sex groups: a 26-year follow-up of the Framingham population. Am Heart J, 111:383-90.

Levy, DE. Bates, D. Caronna, JJ. Cartlidge, NE. Knill-Jones, RP. Lapinski, RH. Singer, BH. Shaw, DA. & Plum, F. (1981). Prognosis in non-traumatic coma. Ann Intern Med, 94(3):293-301.

Mamoli, B., Sluga, E., Zacherl, H., & Gerstenbrand, F. (1977). The apallic syndrome and secondary lesions of peripheral nerves. Monogr Gesamtgeb Psychiatr Psychiatry Ser, 14:214–24.

Monti, MM. Coleman, MR. & Owen, AM. (2009). Neuroimaging and the vegetative state: resolving the behavioural assessment dilemma? Ann N Y Acad Sci, 1157:81-9.

Monti, MM. Laureys, S. & Owen, AM. (2010). The vegetative state. BMJ, 2; 34:c3765.

Monti, MM. Vanhaudenhuyse, A. Coleman, MR. Boly, M. Pickard, JD. Tshibanda, L. Owen, AM. & Laureys, S. (2010). Willful modulation of brain activity in disorders of consciousness. N Engl J Med, 18;362(7):579-89.

Müller-Putz, GR. Klobassa, DS. Pokorny, C. Pichler, G. Erlbeck, H. Real, RGL. Kübler, A. Risetti, M. & Mattia, D. (2012). The auditory P300-based ssBCI: A gateway to minimally conscious patients? Abstract:^{34th}Annual International Conference of the IEEE/EMBS, 4672–4675.

Oder, W. (2004). Prognostic factors in severe traumatic brain injury. Journal of Neurology, Neurosurgery and Psychiatry, 5 (4), 7–22.

Pichler, G., Fazekas, F. (2016). Cardiopulmonary arrest is the most frequent cause of the unresponsive wakefulness syndrome: a prospective population-based cohort study in Austria. Resuscitation, 103;94–98.

Plum, F. & Posner, JB. (1972). The diagnosis of stupor and coma. Contemporary Neurology Series, 10:1–286.

Roslenblath, W. (1899). On a remarkable case of concussion. Dtsch Arch Lin Med, 64:406–24.

Sazbon, L., Costeff, H. & Groswasser, Z. (1992). Epidemiological findings in traumatic post-comatose unawareness. Brain Inj, 6(4):359–62.

Sazbon, L. & Groswasser, Z. (1990). Outcome in 134 patients with prolonged post-traumatic unawareness. 1: parameters determining late recovery of consciousness. J Neurosurg, 72: 75-80.

Schabus, M., Pelika, C., Chwala-Schlege, N., Weilhart, K., Roehm, D., Donis, J., Michitsch, G., Pichler, , G. & Klimesch, W. (2011). Oscillatory brain activity in the vegetative and minimally conscious states during a sentence comprehension task. Functional Neurology, 26(1):31-36

Schnakers, C., Vanhaudenhuyse, A., Giacino, J., Ventura, M., Boly, M., Majerus, S., Moonen, G., & Laureys, S. (2009). Diagnostic accuracy of the vegetative and minimally conscious state: clinical consensus versus standardised neurobehavioural assessment. BMC Neurology, 21;9:35.

Seel, RT. Sherer, M. Whyte, J. Katz, DI. Giacino, JT. Rosenbaum, AM. Hammond, FM. Kalmar, K. Pape, TL. Zafonte, R. Biester, RC. Kaelin, D. Kean, J. & Zasler, N. (2010). Assessment scales for disorders of consciousness: evidence-based recommendations for clinical practice and research. Arch Phys Med Rehabil, 91:1795-1813.

Shaw, LJ. Bairey Merz, CN. Pepine, CJ. Reis, SE. Bittner, V. Kelsey, SF. Olson, M. Johnson, BD. Mankad, S. Sharaf, BL. Rogers, WJ. Wessel, TR. Arant, CB. Pohost, GM. Lerman, A. Quyyumi, AA. & Sopko, G. WISE Investigators (2006). Insights from the NHLBI-Sponsored Women's Ischemia Syndrome Evaluation Study: Part 1: gender differences in traditional and novel risk factors, symptom evaluation and gender-optimised diagnostic strategies. J Am Coll Cardiol, 47(3 Suppl): S4–S20.

Stepan, C. Haidinger, G. & Binder, H. (2004). Prevalence of persistent vegetative state/apallic syndrome in Vienna. Eur Neurol, 11:4861-6.

Swahn, E. (1998). The care of patients with ischaemic heart disease from a gender perspective. Eur Heart J, 19: 1758-65.

The Multi-Society Task Force on PVS. (1994). Medical aspects of the persistent vegetative state (1). New England Journal of Medicine, 330(21): 1499–508.

The Multi-Society Task Force on PVS. (1994). Medical aspects of the persistent vegetative state (2). New England Journal of Medicine, 330(22):1572-9.

Van Erp, WS. et al. The vegetative state/unresponsive wakefulness syndrome: a systematic review of prevalence studies. Eur J Neurol 2014;21:1361-8.

Von Wild, K. In cooperation with the TBI Study Council. (2005). Neurorehabilitation following craniocerebral trauma. Eur J Trauma, 59:345-53.

Von Wild, K., Gerstenbrand, F., Dolce, G., Binder, H., Vos, P., Saltuari, L., Alekseenko, Y., Formisano, R., Ritz, A., Ortega-Suhrkamp, E., Jörg, J., Potapov, A., Leon-Carrion, J., Vilcinis, & R.

Zitnay, GA. (2007). Guidelines for quality management of apallic syndrome/vegetative state. Eur J Trauma Emerg Surg, 3:268-292.

Wilson, FC. Harpur, J. Watson, T. & Morrow, JI. (2002). Vegetative state and minimally responsive patients – regional survey, long-term case outcomes and service recommendations. Neuro Rehabilitation, 17(3):231-6.

Zasler, ND. Giacino, J. & Sandel, ME. (1994). The persistent vegetative state. N Engl J Med, 17;331(20):1381.

Zhuber, K., Salzer, M. & Gerstenbrand, F. (1977). The orthopaedic treatment of patients with apallic syndrome. Monogr Gesamtgeb Psychiatr Psychiatry Ser, 14:208-13.

Internet sources

http://www.neuroreha.at/Phasenmodell.html "Phasenmodel der Neurorehabilitation in Österreich"; (see Table 8)

http://www.statistik.at; (see page 41)

http://www.spitalskompass.at; (see page 42)

http://www.rehakompass.at; (see page 42)

http://www.statistik.at/web_de/statistiken/gesundheit/unfaelle/strassenverkehrsunfaelle/index.html; (see page 62)

GLOSSARY

akinetic mutism	severe motor impairment, whereby those affected do not move (akinesia) and do not speak (mutism). It is believed that perception and memory are usually not impaired
antonym	In linguistics, antonyms are words with opposite meanings. e.g. small and large
ascending reticular formation	A functionally defined area of the brain that controls controls attention

Bulbar brain syndrome	refers to a complex of symptoms that arises when brainstem functions fail and is usually the result of a midbrain syndrome
Dissociative stupor	psychiatric disorder in which voluntary movements, speech and normal responses to light, sound and touch are reduced or completely absent
Extrapyramidal motor function	controls motor processes that do not pass via the pyramidal tract
Falx cerebri	Latin for 'cerebral falx'; formed by the dura mater and separates the two cerebral hemispheres
foraminal Herniation	Intrusion of brain tissue into the foramen magnum as a result of increased intracranial pressure
Frontal lobe syndrome	A complex of symptoms resulting from damage to the frontal lobe. A synonymous term is 'dysexecutive syndrome'
Catatonic stupor	A state of physical rigidity whilst fully conscious, in which movements are not performed at all or only very slowly. Often caused by catatonic schizophrenia
Korsakoff Symptoms	A condition first described by the neurologist Korsakoff, characterised by memory impairment, often associated with a lack of motivation and mood swings
limbic system	A functional unit of the brain responsible for processing emotions and the development of instinctual behaviour. It is also credited with intellectual functions
Midbrain syndrome	Compression of the midbrain resulting from increased pressure within the brain, e.g. due to a haemorrhage or oedema
Panencephalitis	A widespread inflammatory disease of the brain
Penumbra	Latin for 'penumbra'; in the context of a cerebral infarction, this refers to the area immediately adjacent to the central necrotic zone that still contains viable cells

proprioceptive system	Latin *proprius* 'own' and *recipere* 'to receive', refers to the system for perceiving body movement and position in space, or the position of individual body parts in relation to one another
Stretch synergisms	involuntary extension of the limbs in response to external or internal stimuli
Umbra	The centre of a cerebral infarction, consisting of irreversibly damaged brain tissue
Uncus	belonging to the uncus, Latin for 'hook'. This is the hook-shaped, rearwardly curved anterior end of the parahippocampal gyrus, or its continuation, visible on the surface of the temporal lobe
Vulnerability	from the Latin *vulnus*, 'wound'; meaning 'vulnerability' or 'susceptibility'

APPENDIX

Diagnostic criteria for the minimally conscious state (MCS) of the "Aspen Neuro-behavioural Conference Workgroup" (Giacino et al. 2002).

Summary (own translation)

MCS: A state of severely impaired consciousness in which signs of conscious awareness of oneself and/or the environment are present. These signs may not be permanent, but are reproducible or last long enough to distinguish them from reflexive behaviour or random events (e.g. movements).

<u>One or more of the following signs are present</u>:

a) Following simple commands

b) Gestural or verbal responses (yes/no), regardless of accuracy

c) Comprehensible verbalisation

d) Purposeful behaviour (movements or affective behaviour) in environmental stimuli but not as a result of reflexive behaviour:

e.g. situation-appropriate laughter or crying, in response to a corresponding verbal or visual stimulus, but not randomly

e.g. verbal response or gesticulation as a direct reaction to a question

e.g. grasping objects, which suggests a deliberate direction of hand movement and the location of the object

e.g. touching or holding objects, adapting to their size and shape

e.g. eye tracking or sustained fixation in response to movement or stimuli

Emerged from MCS: If a patient recovers from MCS and enters stages with increased levels of consciousness, the boundaries between these stages are arbitrarily defined.

For the definition, <u>at least one of the following abilities</u> must be reliably and consistently present:

a) adequate interactive communication (speaking; correct yes/no code; writing with communication aids)

b) accurate yes/no responses to 6 out of 6 questions regarding situational orientation in 2 consecutive examinations (e.g. “Am I pointing at the ceiling?”)

c) adequate use and handling of two different objects in 2 consecutive assessments (e.g. ‘Are you guiding the comb to the hair or a pencil to the sheet of paper)

The following general points should be taken into account:

1) Sufficient stimulus for maximum arousal response
2) Consideration of impairing conditions (e.g. sedatives, infections)
3) Verbal instructions should not be chosen in such a way that the response could be confused with a reflexive behaviour

4) Motor tasks should be achievable in accordance with the patient's motor abilities or impairments

5) Variations in behavioural responses should be tested using different stimuli

6) Assessment should take place in an environment with as few distractions as possible

7) Reassessments and systematic observations should support the validity of the initial assessment

8) Observations by relatives, carers, etc. should be incorporated into the assessment procedure

Excerpt from the translated CRS-R manual

Coma Recovery Scale Revised AUDITORY

Task		Note	**Points**
Object-related	A: Look at the tennis ball (the cup) B: Look at the pencil <u>or</u> A: Pick up the tennis ball B: Pick up the pencil <u>or</u> A: Kick the ball B: Kick the pencil	(40 cm apart) 10 sec. observation (repeat the instruction once in between) 4 times in total (A-B-A-B)	**4** points (**MCS**) Correct response in all 4 rounds (DG) with at least 2 prompts (=8 in total)
Non-object-related	A: Look away from me B: Look up at the ceiling <u>or</u> A: Touch my hand B: Move a body part <u>or</u> A: Stick out your tongue B: Open your mouth	4 prompts, observing for 15 seconds each	**3** points (**MCS**) 3 out of 4 correct responses to either object-related or non-object-related prompts
Auditory stimulus	Voice or noise for over 5 seconds standing behind the patient; 4 times in total (1st round right–left; 2nd round: right-left)		**2** points Head and/or eye movement towards the stimulus in both directions for at least one direction
Loud noise	Above the patient's head and outside the field of vision; 4 times		**1** point Blink at least twice
Loud noise	See above		**0** points

		No reaction

Excerpt from the translated CRS-R manual

Coma Recovery Scale Revised VISUAL

Task		**Points**
Object recognition	# see auditory (4 trials; A-B-A-B)	**5** points (**MCS**) at least 3 clear responses in 4 trials
Object localisation/ Movement towards the object	Identify the arm or leg with the greatest range of motion; for lower limb, e.g. comb or toothbrush; for upper limb, e.g. ball; present the object approx. 20 cm to the left or right of the limb; Instruction: Touch the object for 10 seconds; repeat the instruction once in between 4 repetitions in total (left-right-left-right) !!! The object does not need to be touched – movement towards it is sufficient!!!	**4** points (**MCS**) – at least 3 clear responses in 4 trials
Eye tracking	Hand mirror: 10–15 cm in front of the face Patient should follow with their gaze: 45° left to right, up to down / 2 times each !!! If negative, then examine with an eye patch; each eye individually!!!	**3** points (**MCS**) 2x eye tracking in any direction
Fixation	Colourful or illuminated object: 15 20 cm in front of the face Movement left-to-right, up-to-down / 4 times in total	**2** points (**MCS**) Fixation for at least 2 seconds > 2 times
Visual Startle response	Move a finger approx. 2.5 cm in front of the eye (without pulling) Open eyes if necessary; 4 times on each eye	**1** point Twitching or blinking at least 2 times
None Startle response	see above	**0** points No reaction

Excerpt from the translated CRS-R manual

Coma Recovery Scale Revised MOTOR SKILLS

Task		**Points**
Functional Use of objects	Place 2 objects (e.g. cup/comb) alternately in the patient's hand and instruct them to demonstrate how to use the object. A-B-A-B	**6** points: **emerged MCS** all 4 trials correct; not possible in cases of paresis

	= 4 trials	
Automated motor response	# Spontaneous motor behaviour (e.g. scratching the nose) # if no spontaneous motor behaviour, then prompt: 1) Show me how to wave 2) I wave, do you not (Demonstrate waving) 2x # If the patient cannot move a limb, use <u>a spoon</u>: 1) Show me how to use the spoon 2) They do not move 2x	**5** points (**MCS**) at least 2x during examination Always waves at 1, but not at 2 Opens mouth only at 1, not at 2
Object manipulation	A tennis ball is rolled over the back of the hand (thumb, index finger). 4 times. Instruction: "Take the ball"	**4** points (**MCS**) In 3 out of 4 cases, the hand is turned and held for at least 5 seconds.
Movement towards the pain stimulus	5 sec. pressure on the most mobile extremity: right hand (fingers or toes) – left hand – right hand – left hand (4 times each)	**3** points (**MCS**) The non-stimulated limb is moved twice and touches the stimulation site
Movement away from the pain	Firm pressure on the nail bed OE right - OE left - UE right - UE left (4 times each)	**2** points: only the stimulated limb moves away from the pain
Pathological pattern	see above (slow, stereotypical flexion of the upper or lower extremity)	**1** point
No reaction, flaccid	See above	**0** points; no response

Excerpt from the translated CRS-R manual

Coma Recovery Scale Revised OROMOTOR / VERBAL

Task		**Points**
Intelligible Verbalisation	1) Tell the patient: "I would like to hear your voice" At least one prompt from the auditory and visual set 2) <u>Auditory set</u>: "What is your name?" or "How are you?" (3 times with a 15-second pause) <u>Visual set:</u> "What is this object called?"	**3** points (**MCS**) All 3 criteria must be met: **1:** Vocalisation must contain K-V-K; e.g. no (e.g. 'nee' is not acceptable) **2:** Two different words; not perfect but understandable. **3:** Words may also be written or displayed on a board .

	(10" on the right and left sides of the screen) or "How many fingers am I holding up?" (1 finger, 10" high)	
Vocalisation / oral movement	Observation of non-reflexive oral movements occurring during the prompts. ! Yawning counts as an oral reflex!	**2** points at least 1x.
Oral reflex	Tongue depressor in mouth	**1** point biting, pumping, chewing
None	See above	**0** points No reaction to any of the stimuli

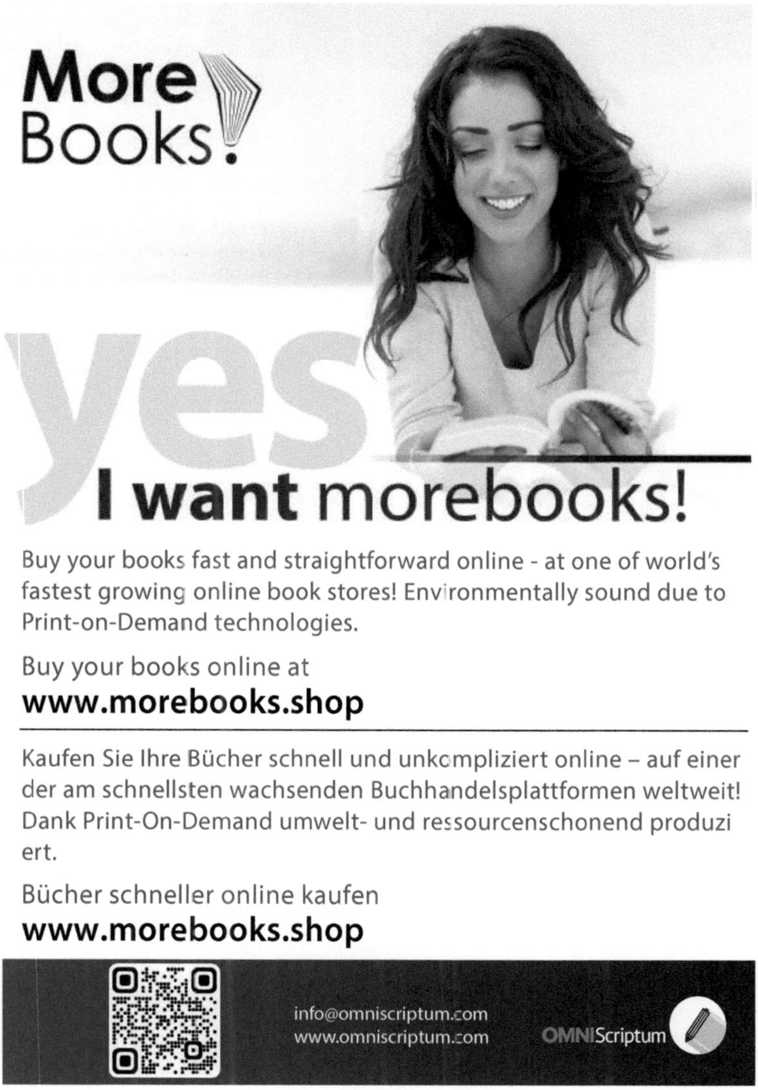
More Books!
yes
I want morebooks!
Buy your books fast and straightforward online - at one of world's fastest growing online book stores! Environmentally sound due to Print-on-Demand technologies.
Buy your books online at
www.morebooks.shop
Kaufen Sie Ihre Bücher schnell und unkompliziert online – auf einer der am schnellsten wachsenden Buchhandelsplattformen weltweit! Dank Print-On-Demand umwelt- und ressourcenschonend produziert.
Bücher schneller online kaufen
www.morebooks.shop
info@omniscriptum.com
www.omniscriptum.com
OMNIScriptum

MIX
Papier aus verantwortungsvollen Quellen
Paper from responsible sources
FSC® C105338

Printed by Books on Demand GmbH, Norderstedt / Germany